Antonia Neumann

Explorations on
Martha Rogers' Science of Unitary Human Beings

Explorations on
Martha Rogers' Science of Unitary Human Beings

Editor

Violet M. Malinski, Ph.D., R.N.
Hunter-Bellevue School of Nursing
Hunter College of the City University of New York
New York, New York

 APPLETON-CENTURY-CROFTS/Norwalk, Connecticut

0-8385-2493-1

Copyright © 1986 by Appleton-Century-Crofts
A Publishing Division of Prentice-Hall

86 87 88 89 90 / 10 9 8 7 6 5 4 3 2 1

Prentice-Hall of Australia, Pty. Ltd., Sydney
Prentice-Hall Canada, Inc.
Prentice-Hall Hispanoamericana, S.A., Mexico
Prentice-Hall of India Private Limited, New Delhi
Prentice-Hall International (UK) Limited, London
Prentice-Hall of Japan, Inc., Tokyo
Prentice-Hall of Southeast Asia (Pte.) Ltd., Singapore
Whitehall Books Ltd., Wellington, New Zealand
Editora Prentice-Hall do Brasil Ltda., Rio de Janeiro

Library of Congress Cataloging-in-Publication Data

Explorations on Martha Rogers' science of unitary human beings.

Includes bibliographies and index.
1. Nursing—Philosophy.   2. Rogers, Martha E.
I. Malinski, Violet M.   II. Title: Unitary human beings.
[DNLM: 1. Philosophy, Nursing. WY 86 E96]
RT84.5.E97   1986   610.73'01   86–14138
ISBN 0–8385–2493–1

Cover: Cindy Lee Lombardo
Design: M. Chandler Martylewski

PRINTED IN THE UNITED STATES OF AMERICA

To Martha E. Rogers for her vision of nursing

Contributors

Martha Raile Alligood, Ph.D., R.N.
Graduate Faculty
University of Florida
Gainesville, Florida
Formerly Director and Associate Professor
Ohio University
Athens, Ohio

Elizabeth Ann Manhart Barrett, Ph.D., R.N.
Assistant Director, Nursing
Mount Sinai Medical Center
Psychotherapist, Private Practice
New York, New York

W. Richard Cowling, III, Ph.D., R.N.
Frances Payne Bolton School of Nursing
Case Western Reserve University
Cleveland, Ohio

Helen M. Ference, Ph.D., R.N.
Private Consultant and Nurse Researcher
Pebble Beach, California

Joyce J. Fitzpatrick, Ph.D., R.N.
Dean and Professor
Frances Payne Bolton School of Nursing
Case Western Reserve University
Cleveland, Ohio

Sarah Hall Gueldner, D.S.N.
Medical College of Georgia
School of Nursing
Athens, Georgia

Sharon F. McDonald, Ph.D., R.N.
Boynton Health Service
University of Minnesota
Minneapolis, Minnesota

Violet M. Malinski, Ph.D., R.N.
Hunter-Bellevue School of Nursing
Hunter College of the City University of New York
New York, New York

Marilyn M. Rawnsley, D.N.Sc.
Professor and Associate Dean for Faculty and Academic Affairs
Lienhard School of Nursing
Pace University
Psychotherapist, Private Practice (Situational Losses)
Pleasantville, New York

Francelyn Reeder, Ph.D., R.S.M., C.N.M.
School of Nursing
University of Colorado
Denver, Colorado

Martha E. Rogers, Sc.D., R.N.
Professor Emeritus
Division of Nursing
New York University
New York, New York

Contents

Preface

The following is a chronological overview of the evolution of the Science of Unitary Human Beings as developed in the major published works of Dr. Martha E. Rogers.[4-12] The references appearing at the end will guide the reader interested in more comprehensive study of this paradigm. Especially noteworthy are the works of Reeder[3] and Sarter.[13] Reeder provides a comprehensive analysis of Rogers' ideas, beginning with her 1961 book, *Educational Revolution in Nursing*. In a conversation with Rogers, Sarter explores the ways in which her ideas have evolved over the years. Critiques of the system can be found in such texts as those by Fawcett[1] and Fitzpatrick.[2]

Martha E. Rogers is an internationally known leader in nursing. She received a diploma in nursing from Knoxville General Hospital and degrees from George Peabody College; Teachers College, Columbia University; and Johns Hopkins University. Rogers was founding executive director of the Visiting Nurse Service in Phoenix, Arizona, an organization she started with two other nurses in 1945. From 1954 to 1975 she headed the Division of Nursing at New York University where she helped to build one of the first Ph.D. programs in nursing. She is now professor emeritus there.

Rogers has long believed that nursing is a learned profession, one that is both a science and an art. A prolific writer and speaker, she has explored a variety of areas ranging from educational preparation, licensure issues, and the nature of nursing science to the current state of the health care system. Her views have often been considered radical by her colleagues.

In *Educational Revolution in Nursing,* Rogers identified the need for a unique nursing science which would serve as the theoretical base for practice. She envisioned this nursing science as one predicated upon holism and the interconnectedness of people and environment. The year 1962 marked the debut of the journal, *Nursing Science,* for which she served as editor.

Turning to the educational preparation of nurses, Rogers presented a rationale for a professional curriculum in nursing in her 1964 book, *Reveille in Nursing*. Baccalaureate programs in nursing would provide the ''cornerstones of nursing's educational system''[5] and the foundation upon which masters and doctoral programs in nursing would build. Nursing science, conceptualized with the person in his or her wholeness and in constant interaction with the universe, "continuous with nature, an open system,"[5] "is directed toward understanding the life process in MAN."[5] *Nursing practice evolving from this scientific base is the process used to assist "human beings to move in the direction of maximum well-being."[5] Nursing, then, is concerned with all people, not just those who are ill.[5]

Rogers explicated this nursing science in her third book, *An Introduction to the Theoretical Basis of Nursing,* published in 1970. Working with her, many doctoral students explored her ideas and conceptualized studies around them. The first doctoral dissertation to test hypotheses derived solely from her system was completed in 1976.

MAJOR WORKS BY MARTHA E. ROGERS, 1967–1985

1967. In a paper presented at the Annual Conference on Research and Nursing at Teachers College, entitled "Nursing Science: Research and Researchers," Rogers elaborated on her view of nursing as a learned profession with two dimensions, the science of nursing and the use of this knowledge for the betterment of "man." Professional education in nursing represents the transmission of a body of abstract principles arrived at by research and logical analysis rather than technical skills. This nursing science describes, explains, and predicts the life process. She further identified "man," the phenomenon of concern to nursing, as an integrated whole, a living system that

- is a complex electro-dynamic field (later changed to an energy field)
- is an open system
- is unidirectional (later changed to four dimensional)
- maintains pattern amidst constant change (first changed to "is identified by pattern and organization"[5] then modified to the word "patterning" in a move away from static connotation of the earlier wording).

1970. Rogers' text, *An Introduction to the Theoretical Basis of Nursing,* is organized into three units. In the first unit, she provided an historical perspective on culture, modern science, and evolutionary thought as a background for modern nursing. In the second, she specified the phenomenon of "man" as a unified whole, an open system, and a sentient, thinking being. Rogers went on to discuss the unidirectionality and pattern and organization of life. In the third unit, she presented the conceptual system including the Principles of Homeodynamics, broad generalizations which she offered as conforming to experiential data and which would lay the foundation for developing testable hypotheses. There were four at the time:

---

* Rogers has responded to the call for non-sexist language and now uses the term "unitary human being" rather than "man" or "unitary man."

1. *Principle of reciprocy:* "postulates the inseparability of man and environment and predicts that sequential changes in the life process are continuous, probabilistic revisions occurring out of the interactions between man and environment" (p. 97).[7]
2. *Principle of synchrony:* "change in the human field depends only upon the state of the human field and the simultaneous state of the environmental field at any given point in space–time" (p. 98).[7]
3. *Principle of helicy:* "the life process evolves unidirectionally in sequential stages along a curve which has the same general shape all along but which does not lie in a plane. Encompassed within this principle are the concepts of rhythmicality, negentropic evolutionary emergence, and the unitary nature of the man–environment relationship" (p. 99).[7] Rogers noted that helicy subsumed within it reciprocy and synchrony.
4. *Principle of resonancy:* "change in pattern and organization of the human field and the environmental field is propagated by waves" (p. 101).[7] In describing waves, Rogers noted, "Light waves, sound waves, thermal waves, atomic waves, gravity waves, flow in rhythmic patterns—largely unseen, unheard, and unopen to man's capacity to see, hear, or perceive."[7]

In summing up the importance of the Principles of Homeodynamics, Rogers noted that they provide a way of perceiving "unitary man." Changes in man are inseparable from changes in the environment, reflecting the mutual, simultaneous interaction of the two. Changes are irreversible, nonrepeating, and rhythmical, proceeding via resonating waves of growing complexity of pattern and organization. She shared beginning insights into the ways in which the conceptual system could be translated into practice, citing studies conducted by doctoral students at New York University examining such variables as rocking and motion. In conclusion, Rogers called for a design for relevance, "a constructive approach to achieving human health and welfare," based on a philosophy of life's creativity and a belief in our evolutionary future, noting that "a design for relevance requires the seeing of a pattern."[7]

1980. In the decade between the publication of her textbook and her next published work, the system underwent considerable refinement. For example, Rogers dropped the principles of synchrony and reciprocy, maintaining that they were subsumed under helicy. In addition, these two principles had created confusion, as people were interpreting them using definitions outside the system. This modification appeared in print in 1980[8] along with the addition of complementarity, the continuous, mutual, simultaneous interaction of human and environmental fields, as the third principle (later changed to integrality).

Rogers again identified the focus of nursing, "unitary man," as distinctive to nursing. She defined the science of nursing as one that "seeks to study the nature and direction of unitary human development integral with the environment and to evolve the descriptive, explanatory, and predictive principles basic to knowledge-able practice."[8] The four building blocks were identified as

1. energy fields
2. openness
3. pattern and organization
4. four dimensionality, postulating a world with neither space nor time, rather than the original "space–time," with the idea of a "relative present" rather than the present as a point in time.[8]

Noting that theories are derived from a conceptual system, Rogers briefly described three such derivations:

1. *Theory of accelerating evolution:* accelerating change is characterized by higher wave frequency pattern and organization, with implications for understanding such clinical phenomena as hyperactivity and hypertension.
2. *Paranormal events:* the relative present is different for each human being, an idea having implications for explaining clairvoyance, precognition, and similar phenomena.
3. *Rhythmical correlates of change:* human rhythms, perceived as field behaviors, are manifestations of the whole. For example, the sleep–wake pattern can be seen as an indication of evolutionary emergence from sleeping, to waking, to beyond waking.[8]

1981–1982. Rogers presented her ideas at the International Congress on Applied Systems Research and Cybernetics in Mexico in a paper entitled, "Science of Unitary Man: A Paradigm for Nursing." She discussed manifestations of change, a speeding up of human rhythms which she saw as coordinate with higher frequency environmental patterns. She presented a new view of aging within this perspective as opposed to the traditional view of aging as one of decay and running down. Rogers also highlighted the implications of four dimensionality for alternative healing modalities such as therapeutic touch and meditation. In another work[10], Rogers described her vision of the future, again dealing with such issues as nursing education and the health care system as a medical monopoly.

1983. Rogers addressed the concept of the family within what she was now identifying as a paradigm rather than a conceptual system, noting that the Science of Unitary Human Beings (no longer identified as the Science of Unitary Man) is equally applicable to families as to individual human beings. "An irreducible, four dimensional, negentropic family energy field becomes the focus of study."[11] Rogers saw the term "family" as applying to a broad range of possible configurations of which the traditional nuclear family is only one example. Manifestations of the family–environment interaction process, such as sleep–wake patterns of the family and rhythmical correlates of activity, could be observed as indices of the family.

Year	Chapter	Researcher	School	Variables	Science of Unitary Human Beings Principles	Design	Support for Hypotheses
1977	8	Rawnsley	Boston University	Time experienced; State of human energy field (dying, not dying); Age (younger, older)	Principles	Descriptive (four groups)	Partial
1979	9	Ference	New York University	Time experience; Creativity traits; Differentiation; Human field motion—tool developed and tested	Resonancy	Correlational (canonical) Methodological	Yes
1980	10	Malinski	New York University	Hyperactivity; Color preference; Vision along the short wavelength end of the spectrum	Theory of Accelerating Evolution	Correlational	No
1981	11	McDonald	Wayne State	Visible lightwaves (blue, red, control); Presence/absence of a visual barrier; Duration of exposure; Pain perception	Rhythm Theory	Mixed Experimental	Partial
1982	12	Cowling	New York University	Mystical experience; Differentiation; Creativity	Helicy	Correlational	Yes
1982	13	Alligood	New York University	Creativity; Actualization; Empathy	Helicy	Correlational	Yes
1983	14	Gueldner	University of Alabama	Imposed motion (rocking); Human field motion; Restedness	Resonancy	Quasi-Experimental	Partial
1983	15	Barrett	New York University	Human field motion—devised a new method of analyzing and scoring; Power—scales developed and tested	Helicy	Methodological Correlational (canonical)	Yes

Rogers stated, "The integrality of people with environment, coordinate with a universe of open systems, identifies the scope of a paradigm for nursing."[11] This use of "integrality" signaled the coming change from complementarity to the principle of integrality. This change was not made explicit until Rogers' paper, "Science of Unitary Human Beings: A Paradigm for Nursing," written in 1983. This paper can be found in the monograph, *Examining the Cultural Implications of Martha E. Rogers' Science of Unitary Human Beings*.[12] Further explication of Rogers' work can be found in Chapters 1 and 2 of the present text.

This book arises from a network of people who conducted basic research within the Science of Unitary Human Beings. Studies derived from this conceptual system are presented to the reader in the spirit in which they were undertaken— the spirit of inquiry. We wanted to share our experiences in conducting research, successes and misses, in the hope of stimulating further dialogue into research within this conceptual system.

All of the studies were undertaken as doctoral dissertations. Many of the contributors had the opportunity to work with Martha Rogers in some phase of their work. Five contributors did their doctoral work at New York University, one at Boston University, one at Wayne State University, and one at the University of Alabama at Birmingham. Marilyn Rawnsley was the first person to do doctoral research totally within this conceptual system.

The studies were completed between 1976 and 1983. They are arranged chronologically and reflect changes in Rogers' conceptualization and terminology over the years, a reflection of the dynamic nature of this system. Contributors were asked to present their work within the original conceptualizations of the studies rather than from an updated perspective. They complied with space limitations in presenting their work and therefore left much unwritten. Interested readers are referred to the appropriate dissertations for complete discussions.

I hope this book will contribute to networking among those nurses who are interested in the Science of Unitary Human Beings. It should provide a frame work to facilitate an exchange of ideas with colleagues.

REFERENCES

1. Fawcett J: Analysis and Evaluation of Conceptual Models of Nursing. Philadelphia, FA Davis, 1984
2. Fitzpatrick J, Whall A: Conceptual Models of Nursing: Analysis and Application. Bowie, Md, Robert J Brady, 1983
3. Reeder F: Nursing Research, Holism and Philosophies of Science: Points of Congruence Between E Husserl and ME Rogers, doctoral dissertation. New York University, 1984 (University Microfilms Publication No. 84–21, 466)
4. Rogers ME: Educational Revolution in Nursing. New York, MacMillan Company, 1961

5. Rogers ME: Reveille in Nursing. Philadelphia: FA Davis, 1964
6. Rogers ME: Nursing science: Research and researchers. In Teachers College Report. New York, Teachers College, 1967.
7. Rogers ME: An Introduction to the Theoretical Basis of Nursing. Philadelphia: FA Davis, 1970
8. Rogers ME: Nursing: A science of unitary man. In Riehl JP, Roy C (eds): Conceptual Models for Nursing Practice, 2nd ed. New York, Appleton-Century-Crofts, 1980, 329–337
9. Rogers ME: Science of unitary man: A paradigm for nursing. In Laskar GE (ed): Applied Systems and Cybernetics, Vol. IV. New York, Pergamon, 1981
10. Rogers ME: Beyond the horizon. In Chaska N (ed): The Nursing Profession: A Time to Speak. New York, McGraw-Hill, 1982, pp. 795–801
11. Rogers ME: Science of unitary human beings: A paradigm for nursing. In Clements IW, Roberts FB (eds): Family Health: A Theoretical Approach to Nursing Care. New York, Wiley, 1983, pp. 219–228
12. Rogers ME: Science of unitary human beings: A paradigm for nursing. In Wood R, Kekahbah, J (eds): Examining the Cultural Implications of Martha E. Rogers' Science of Unitary Human Beings. Lecompton, Kansas, Wood-Kekahbah Associates, 1985
13. Sarter B: The Stream of Becoming: A Metaphysical Analysis of Rogers' Model of Unitary Man, doctoral dissertation. New York University, 1984 (University Microfilms)

Acknowledgments

Grateful acknowledgment is made for permission to reproduce the following:

From *Order Out of Chaos* by Ilya Prigogine and Isabelle Stengers. Copyright (c) 1984. By permission of Bantam Books, Inc. All rights reserved.

From *Mind and Nature: A Necessary Unity* by Gregory Bateson. Copyright (c) 1979. By permission of E. P. Dutton, Inc.

From "Morphogenetic Fields and the Implicate Order" by David Bohm and Rupert Sheldrake, 1982. By permission of *ReVision Journal*.

From "The Problem of Proof" by Ken Wilber, 1982. By permission of *ReVision Journal*.

From *The Tao of Physics* by Fritjof Capra. Copyright (c) 1975, 1983. Reprinted with permission of Shambhala Publications, Inc., Boulder, Colorado.

Introduction

Joyce J. Fitzpatrick

Science, according to Rogers, is an organized body of abstract knowledge arrived at by scientific research and logical analysis. The nursing perspective specifies the body of scientific knowledge basic to nursing. The art of nursing is the imaginative and creative use of nursing knowledge in human service.

Rogers' vision of nursing has been a guiding force for nearly two decades. Her professional and scholarly influence has been strong. She has led her colleagues and students to new understandings and explications of the nursing reality. Her work has strengthened nursing education, leadership, science, and professional practice.

The Science of Unitary Human Beings has been presented by Rogers as a paradigm for nursing. The paradigm has guided the research of the authors who contributed chapters in this book. The development of these scientists as a community of scholars has been further enhanced by this synthesis, the elaboration here of the central themes in the conceptualization and empirical testing of theoretical postulations.

One frequent concern that has previously been expressed about Rogers' model is that it is not testable. At times this has been further translated to a lack of precise operational definitions and specific hypotheses. Rogers' conceptualization includes multiple theories which may be subjected to empirical test. Much evidence of that testing is presented here.

Rogers' conceptualization can be reviewed according to the characteristics of sound conceptual or theoretical systems. The specific criteria include: (1) explicit boundaries, (2) congruence with empirical evidence, (3) generality, (4) usefulness, (5) significance, (6) capability of generating hypotheses, (7) internal consistency, and (8) simplicity or parsimony.

First, Rogers' scientific model has explicit boundaries. The approach to science development in nursing, aside from Rogers' model, has been largely additive. The belief prevails that yes, nurses study holistic persons, and the way to specify that holistic view is to add the parts. So a little, or a lot, depending on one's orientation and educational background, of the ingredients of the psychological, sociological, physiological, biological, and sometimes, spiritual, perspective *and* a synthesis of these leads one to nursing knowledge. The pragmatists among us, however, would propose that the synthesis is not critical, but rather nursing knowledge is derived from the application of knowledge from other sciences to nursing situations. The additive approach to knowledge development usually is accompanied by a reductionistic scientific method. Proponents advocate reducing the whole to its smallest parts, studying these parts, and then inferring about the whole.

Rogers advocates studying the whole. She argues against reductionism and encourages the development of new scientific approaches to basic nursing questions. Some knowledge is excluded due to the explicit conceptual boundaries. Kuhn[2] has well described the fallacy of our belief in a science which is cumulative in nature. Science does not tend toward this ideal image; rather new scientific paradigms, while arising from the old, replace old paradigms. Therefore, some knowledge systems necessarily will be excluded by the new boundaries.

Second, a conceptual or theoretical system should be congruent with empirical evidence. A second related fallacy in our beliefs about science is the assumption that paradigms and theories are either true or false. We are often in search of the ideal truth. Rather, we must ask ourselves to what extent paradigms and theories are adequate or inadequate in explaining the world or the phenomena of concern. They must be more or less consistent with what is known, with the accumulated empirical evidence. Kuhn[2] described the logical fallacy of belief that one can ever purely verify or falsify through the development of science. Rather, science is an approximation of reality, a search for truth, but a search cognizant of the unreachable goal. The predominant scientific view is that which does the best job of explaining the phenomena of concern.

Arguments regarding relevance of a scientific perspective have centered around the generality, the usefulness, and the significance of conceptual or theoretical systems (criteria three, four, and five). What if these three additional criteria are applied to the Science of Unitary Human Beings? Does this conceptualization possess generality? Again, here the strength of the conceptualization is the component that has been highly criticized. For it is the abstract nature of conceptualizations of energy fields, four dimensionality, and wave patterns that lead pragmatists to become skeptical, and ask: "How can I nurse an energy field?" One *can* provide nursing care to persons while understanding the abstract conceptualizations of energy fields. Is this conceptual system useful? And of course one must ask, useful for what? For detailing nursing interventions? For providing checklists for tracking nursing activities? For prescribing interventions? If the belief is held that nursing science must strive toward prescriptive theory, then one will remain skeptical of a world view that proposes development of basic knowledge of persons as fundamental for nursing science. Is this conceptual system significant? Judging the number of related theoretical developments, and the applications in both research and in professional practice, one must conclude that this scientific development has had a marked impact on the further development of nursing science.

A sixth criterion to judge the adequacy of a conceptual or theoretical model is its capabiltiy of generating hypotheses. Rogers' conceptualization has consistently generated hypotheses for testing, some of which have been more directly linked and logically consistent with the basic assumptions underlying the conceptualization. The evidence gathered here will add to the further development of Rogers' conceptualization.

The seventh criterion is that of internal consistency. All analyses of Rogers' conceptualizaiton support the basic inherent logic and consistency. Rogers does not waver. Systems are not a little bit closed, and persons are not sometimes whole.

The last criterion to be addressed here is that of simplicity or parsimony. Science is the search for simplicity. William of Occam, a 14th century philosopher, said, "Entities should not be multiplied beyond necessity." This principle of parsimony means that no more forces should be postulated than are necessary to account for the phenomenon observed. In practice, this means that the simplest explanation is the best. Rogers' conceptualization, even in its complexity in terminology and essence, has a simplicity in form and structure.

This manuscript represents an extension of Rogers' work in the development of nusing science. In the Preface, Malinski presents an overview of the Science to Unitary Human Beings developed by Rogers. This serves as a good orientation to the chapters that follow. In chapter 1 Rogers presents her basic conceptual system. This is a necessary introduction. In Chapters 2, 3, and 4 Malinski sets the stage for the research to be presented. These chapters alone present significant new views on Rogers' conceptualization. The conversation with Rogers in Chapter 2 is particularily useful to those who have not had such conversations. Rogers' own humanness is apparent here as she responds to questions and further elaborates the essential components of her view. Malinski's explication of the parallels between contemporary science and nursing science is an important contribution to scholarship. The works of Capra, Bohm, and Prigogine should become familiar to all students of Rogers and all scholars in nursing. Malinski's contribution to relevance for practice of Rogers' work, as presented in Chapter 4, may be the most remembered and the most remarkable. Practicing nurses everywhere have been searching for some of these relationships. Chapter 5 includes Ference's statements regarding the evolution of nursing science. She presents an historical perspective of science development as related to Rogers' conceptualization. In Chapter 6 Reeder explicates basic theoretical research in this conceptual system. She recommends further study from a phenomenological perspective.

Cowling's work presented in Chapter 7, on the theoretical issues, methodological challenges, and research realities related to this science is particularly instructive. He sets the stage for the specific studies presented in the following chapters. He presents a excellent summary of the important questions facing each researcher working within Rogers' area of knowledge development.

The chapters that follow each include a presentation of a specific study based on Rogers' conceptualizaiton. These range from the study completed by Rawnsley in 1977 to the 1983 studies of Gueldner and Barrett. All of these were undertaken as dissertation research; four different universities provided the sites for doctoral study for them.

Rawnsley's study was one of younger and older persons, some of whom were dying and some of whom were not dying. She was concerned with the state of the energy field during this dying experience and with all of the principles included in Rogers' conceptualization. The specific variable measured was that of time perception.

Ference also studied time expeience, but identified additional variables of creativity and field differentiation as related to Rogers' science. The basic interest of the Ference study was human field motion. Ference developed and tested a human field motion instrument derived from her understanding of the principle of resonancy.

Malinski investigated the relationship between color and hyperactivity, based on a theory of accelerating evolution. She was particularly concerned with vision along the short wave length end of the color spectrum.

McDonald's study was also focused on light waves, in this case the visible waves of blue, red, and white. She studied their relationship to pain perception with arthritic persons experiencing chronic pain based on rhythm theory.

Cowling studied the relationships between mystical experience, creativity, and differentiation. He was interested in further explications based on the helicy principle.

Alligood also explicated relationships based on the helicy principle. Variables included were creativity, actualization, and empathy.

Gueldner placed older persons in rocking chairs and used imposed motion to study its relationship to human field motion and restedness. Gueldner elaborated her study based on the principle of resonancy.

Barrett also studied human field motion related to the principle of helicy. She included a major instrument development component and introduced the variable of power related to Rogers' science.

These studies are all evidence of new realities in nursing research. Why have nurses, scientists, researchers, and practitioners been so reluctant to embrace this new vision of reality? Basically, because it is hard to change. As a group we have invested large amounts of time and energy, and particularly thought, in our current conceptualizations and in their confirmation through a predominant scientific mode rooted in empiricism. Only recently have we begun to question the inherent values of the scientific paradigm of empiricism.[4,6] Others have recommended that we embrace all scientific approaches in our quest for knowledge development in nursing.[1,5] And, of course, more extreme positions have been advanced, i.e., that scientific methods, in and of themselves, are not compatible with an humanistic holistic perspective of humans.[3] Most critical it would seem in this scientific development of nursing are the answers to the questions: What are the phenomena of concern to nursing? What are the specific questions that nursing must address as a discipline? Theoretical developments based on Rogers' conceptualization must be logically consistent with the basic concepts and principles. For example, based on Rogers' descriptions of energy fields characterized by wholeness and wave patterns there has been a significant body of nursing research regarding rhythmic phenomena. Analysis of the theoretical derivations and the operationalization of concepts is necessary to judge the logical consistency of these studies with Rogers' conceptualization. Nevertheless, the attempt has been made to further explicate the model, to derive testable theorems, to test empirically the derived hypotheses, and even to further refine the basic conceptualizations. In support of Rogers' scientific developments it is also instructive to attend to scientific process. Gortner[1] has aptly described the development of a scientific ethos in nursing based on four principles of scientific work: confirmation, communality, competition and colleagueship, and continuity. Rogers has fostered these principles in her scientific pursuits and those of her colleagues and students. She has fostered dialogue and communication with and among others to develop a community of scholars. Rogers has encouraged both competition and colleagueship as evidenced by graduates of educational programs she developed, and she has advocated programmatic research efforts related to the Science of Unitary Human Beings. Rogers' science has been exemplary in these dimensions. This book is a major extension of that contribution.

REFERENCES

1. Gortner S: Nursing science in transition. Nurs Res 29:180–183, 1980
2. Kuhn T: The Structure of Scientific Revolutions, 2nd ed. Chicago, University of Chicago Press, 1970
3. Munhall PL: Nursing philosophy and nursing research: In apposition or opposition? Nurs Res 3:176–177, 181, 1982
4. Tinkle MB, Beaton JL: Toward a new view of science: Implications for nursing research. Adv in Nrsg Sci 5:27–36, January, 1983
5. Walker LO, Avant KC: Strategies for Theory Construction in Nursing. Norwalk, Conn, Appleton-Century-Crofts, 1983
6. Winstead-Fry P: The scientific method and its impact on holistic health. Adv in Nrsg Sci 2:1–7, July, 1980

Explorations
on
Martha Rogers'
Science of Unitary
Human Beings

Part One

The Paradigm

1

Science of Unitary Human Beings

Martha E. Rogers

Some years ago Elizabeth Kemble* pointed out that ". . . much has been written and said concerning the spirit, art, and science of nursing. No one will deny the importance of all three in the effective practice of nursing. But the noble spirit alone is not enough. The art of nursing falls short even with a fine spirit. It is only when nursing practice is based on a theoretically sound foundation that the spirit and art can come into full being." The theoretically sound foundation that gives identity to nursing as a science and an art requires an organized abstract system from which to derive unifying principles and hypothetical generalizations. Through basic and applied research, principles and theories are tested. New understandings emerge. New questions arise. Description, explanation, and prediction take on new meanings. A substantive body of knowledge specific to nursing takes form.

The uniqueness of nursing, like that of any other science, lies in the phenomenon central to its purpose. Nursing's long-established concern with human beings and their world is a natural forerunner of an organized abstract system encompassing people and their environments. The irreducible nature of individuals as energy fields, different from the sum of their parts and integral with their respective environmental fields, differentiates nursing from other sciences and identifies nursing's focus.

A Science of Unitary Human Beings basic to nursing requires a new world view and a conceptual system specific to nursing phenomena of concern. The development of a science portends the emergence of abstract concepts and a corresponding language of specificity. Scientific language evolves out of the general

---

* Former Dean of the University of North Carolina School of Nursing at Chapel Hill, N.C.

language. Terms specific to the system are defined for clarity and precision. Uniformity of usage provides for communication. Rigorous research can be pursued and replicated. All terms, except those defined specific to the system, are interpreted in their general language meaning.

When nursing is perceived as a science, the term *nursing* becomes a noun signifying a body of knowledge. The education of nurses has identity in the transmission of nursing's body of theoretical knowledge. The practice of nursing is the creative use of this knowledge for human betterment. Research in nursing is the study of unitary human beings integral with their environment.

Science is open-ended. Change is continuous. New knowledge brings new insights. The development of a Science of Unitary Human Beings is a never-ending process. The conceptual system first presented some years ago has gained in substance. Concomitantly, errors have undergone correction, definitions have been revised for greater clarity and accuracy, and updating of content is continuous. Basic theoretical research is essential for ongoing development of this field of study.

The development of a conceptual system is a process of creative synthesis of facts and ideas out of which a new product emerges. Principles and theories derive from the system and are tested in the real world. The findings of research are fed back into the system, whereby the system undergoes continuous alteration, revision, and change. A conceptual system exists only in its entirety. It bespeaks wholeness and unity. It provides a way of perceiving people and their world.

The conceptual system that underwrites a Science of Unitary Human Beings does not derive from one or more of the basic sciences. Neither does it come out of a vacuum. A multiplicity of knowledges from many sources flows in novel ways to create a kaleidoscope of potentialities. Fundamental concepts are identified. Significant terms are defined congruent with the evolving system. A humane and optimistic view of life's potentials grows as a new reality appears. People's capacity to participate knowingly in the process of change is postulated.

Unitary human beings are specified to be irreducible wholes. A whole cannot be understood when it is reduced to its particulars. The use of the term *unitary* human beings is not to be confused with current popular usage of the term *holistic,* generally signifying a summation of parts, whether few or many. The unitary nature of environment is equally irreducible. The concept of *field* provides a means of perceiving people and their respective environments as irreducible wholes.

Four concepts are postulated to be basic to the proposed system, namely: energy fields, openness, pattern, and four-dimensionality. These concepts are defined consistent with the general language and are given specificity according to the conceptual system under discussion.

Energy fields are postulated to constitute the fundamental unit of both the living and the nonliving. *Field* is a unifying concept. *Energy* signifies the dynamic nature of the field. *Energy fields* are infinite. Two energy fields are identified: the human field and the environmental field. Specifically, human beings and environment *are* energy fields. They do not have them. Moreover, human and environmental fields are *not* biological fields or physical fields, or social or psychological fields. Neither are human and environmental fields a summation of biological, physical, social, and psychological fields. This is not a denial of other fields. Rather, it is to make clear that human and environmental fields have their own identity and are not to be confused with parts.

A universe of open systems has been gaining support for three-quarters of a century. With introduction of relativity, quantum theory, and probability, the prevailing absolutism, already shaken by evolutionary theory, received a critical blow. By the 1920s Selye was proposing adaptation, and by the 1930s Bertalanffy introduced the idea of negative entropy. Soon Cannon advanced the idea of homeostasis. Space exploration began in the 1950s, and by the 1960s some physiologists suggested replacing the term *homeostasis* with the term *homeokinesis*. As new knowledge escalated, the traditional meanings of *homeostasis, steady-state, adaptation,* and *equilibrium* were no longer tenable. The closed-system, entropic model of the universe began to be questioned.

In a universe of open systems, causality is not an option. Acausality had come in with quantum theory. Bertrand Russell, some years later, noted, "The law of causality . . . is a relic of a bygone age, surviving, like the monarchy, only because it is erroneously supposed to do no harm."[1] Energy fields are open—not a little bit or sometimes, but continuously. The human and environmental fields are integral with one another. Causality is invalid. Change is continuously innovative.

Pattern is defined as the distinguishing characteristic of an energy field perceived as a single wave. Pattern is an abstraction. It gives identity to the field. The nature of the pattern changes continuously. Each human field pattern is unique and is integral with its own unique environmental field pattern. The term "pattern" is used only to refer to an energy field. Manifestations of field pattern emerge out of the human and environmental field mutual process and will be discussed later in this chapter.

Four-dimensionality characterizes the human and environmental fields. It is defined as a nonlinear domain without spatial or temporal attributes. All reality is postulated to be four-dimensional. The relative nature of change becomes explicit. Four-dimensionality is postulated to be a given of this system. It is not something one moves into or becomes. It is a way of perceiving human beings and their world.

Definitions increase in clarity and specificity as the conceptual system emerges. The unitary human being (human field) is defined as an irreducible, four-dimensional energy field identified by pattern and manifesting characteristics that are different from those of the parts and cannot be predicted from knowledge of the parts. The environmental field is defined as an irreducible, four-dimensional energy field identified by pattern and manifesting characteristics different from those of the parts. Each environmental field is specific to its given human field. Both change continuously, mutually, and creatively. The human and environmental fields are infinite and integral with one another.

Unifying principles and hypothetical generalizations derive from the conceptual system. The Principles of Homeodynamics are three in number and together postulate the nature and direction of change. These principles are set forth as follows:

PRINCIPLES OF HOMEODYNAMICS

Principle of Resonancy   The continuous change from lower to higher frequency wave patterns in human and environmental fields

Principle of Helicy   The continuous, innovative, probabilistic increasing diversity of human and environmental field patterns characterized by nonrepeating rhythmicities

Principle of Integrality*   The continuous mutual human field and environmental field process

Pattern is a key concept in these principles. The principles are stated so that they are mutually exclusive, to avoid the confusion that attended earlier definitions. The term *integrality* has replaced *complementarity* to gain greater accuracy and clarity of meaning.

Pattern was noted earlier to be an abstraction. Manifestations of field patterning are observable events in the real world. They are postulated to emerge out of the human–environmental field mutual process. Change is continuous, relative, and innovative. Increasing diversity of field patterning characterizes the process of change. Individual differences point up the significance of relative diversity. For example, changing rhythmicities possess individual uniqueness. Transition from longer sleeping to longer waking to beyond waking is highly variable between individuals. Moreover, further diversity is being manifest in so-called 'day people' and 'night people' as well as in other examples of rhythmical diversity.

Investigations testing the validity of the Principles of Homeodynamics and the postulated nature of change in field pattern manifestations appear in this text. Research in this area is ongoing.

A science has many theories. As these are tested, some will be supported; others may not. Replication of research may contribute to the level of confidence one may have in a given theory. Everyday events, when examined from a new world view, a different perspective, raise new questions and suggest new explanations.

A theory of accelerating evolution deriving from this conceptual system requires a fresh look at today's rapidly changing norms in blood pressure levels, children's behavior, longer waking periods, and other events. Higher frequency wave patterns of growing diversity portend new norms coordinate with accelerating change. Labels of pathology based on old norms generate hypochondriasis— not uncommonly iatrogenic in origin. ''Normal'' means ''average.'' Normal (average) blood pressure readings in all age groups are notably higher today than they were a few decades ago. Evidence that these norms are jeopardizing the public's health is insubstantial. The relative nature of multiplying individual differences in

---

* Formerly titled Principle of Complementarity.

a dynamic, continuously innovative system raises critical questions about the meaning of mass surveys and unrestrained encouragement of frequent blood pressure checks. Drugs are dispensed with largesse and not infrequently cause something less than healthy side effects. Health personnel have long deplored public failure to follow up on recommended "expert" treatment. Could it be that there is a folk wisdom that protects the unwary and the "doubting Thomases"?

Not only has the average waking period lengthened, but sleep–wake continuities are increasingly diverse. Developmental norms have changed significantly in recent years. Gifted children and the so-called hyperactive not uncommonly manifest similar behaviors. It would seem more reasonable to hypothesize hyperactivity as accelerating evolution than to denigrate rhythmicities that diverge from outdated norms and erroneous expectations.

Manifestations of a speeding up of human field rhythms are coordinate with higher frequency environmental field patterns. Radiation increments of widely diverse frequencies are common household accompaniments of everyday life. Atmospheric and cosmological complexity grows. Environmental motion has quickened. A very high-speed transit tube craft that can whisk people across the country by electromagnetic waves at approximately 14,000 miles per hour is already within man's capability. Moon villages and space towns are on the near horizon.

Human and environmental fields evolve together, integral with one another. The doomsayers who predict man's early self-destruction fail to recognize the innovative potentials that abound. Increased longevity, escalating science and technology, outer-space exploration, aroused concern for human rights, and multiple other evidences of man's evolutionary potentials in process of actualization bespeak a future people have scarcely envisioned.

With increased longevity, growing numbers of older persons are added to the population. Contrary to a static view engendered by a closed-system model of the universe, which postulates aging to be a running down, the Science of Unitary Human Beings postulates aging to be a developmental process. Aging is continuous from conception through the dying process. Field patterns are increasingly diverse and creative. The aged sleep less, and sleep–wake frequencies are more varied. Higher frequency patterns give meaning to multiple reports of time experienced as racing.

Aging is not a disease, nor is it analogous to the "one-hoss shay" of literary lore. Innovative developmental diversity manifests itself nonlinearly and in contradiction to the traditional emphasis on chronological age as a determinant in change. More diverse field patterns change more rapidly than the less diverse. Populations defy so-called normal curves as individual differences multiply. This conceptual system predicates a clearly different approach to the aged. Values are revised. A new sense of self-worth becomes evident among older people.

The emergence of paranormal phenomena as valid subjects for serious scientific research has nonetheless been handicapped by a paucity of viable theories to explain these events. The conceptual system presented here provides a framework for generating and testing viable theories. Some are reported in this volume. Alternative forms of healing, meditative modalities, and imagery are increasingly popular. The efficacy of Therapeutic Touch, developed by Dolores Krieger, has been documented. The implications for creative health services are notable. Noninvasive therapies and diminished use of drugs can be expected to replace the current mechanistic emphasis in treating human ills.

Nurses are concerned with the dying as well as with the living. Unitary human and environmental rhythms find expression in the rhythmicities of the living–dying process. Just as aging is deemed developmental, so too is dying hypothesized to be developmental. The nature of the dying process and after-death phenomena have gained considerable public and professional interest in recent years. Investigations into the nature and validity of a range of phenomena associated with dying are reported in the literature. Definitions of death are increasingly arguable. Questionable practices in securing organs for transplantation have led to legislative action. The right to die with dignity is being written into final testaments and debated in courts of law. Concomitantly, reports of near-death and after-death experiences are already listed among the best-sellers. A new approach to studying the dying process is provided by the conceptual system herein presented. The nature and continuity of field patterning subsequent to dying, while admittedly a difficult area to study, nonetheless is open to theoretical investigation.

Research findings support the nature of change postulated in the Principles of Homeodynamics. Some are reported in this book. Others have been completed or are nearing completion. New tools of measurement are necessary adjuncts to studying questions arising out of a world view that is different from the prevalent view. The research potentials of this system are infinite. It is logically and scientifically tenable. It is flexible and open-ended. Practical implications for human betterment are demonstrable.

Seeing the world from this viewpoint requires a new synthesis, a creative leap, and the inculcation of new attitudes and values. Guiding principles are broad generalizations that require imaginative and innovative modalities for their implementation. The Science of Unitary Human Beings identifies nursing's uniqueness and signifies the potential of nurses to fulfill their social responsibility in human service. Basic theoretical research in the Science of Unitary Human Beings is indispensable. Only then can the theoretically sound foundation continue to evolve.

REFERENCE

1. Russell B: On the notion of cause, with applications to the free-will problem. In Feigl H, Brodbeck M (eds): Readings in the Philosophy of Science. New York, Appleton-Century-Crofts, 1953, p 387

2

Further Ideas from Martha Rogers

Violet M. Malinski

In an effort to facilitate the reader's comprehension of this conceptual system, the following discussion synthesizes ideas pertinent to Rogers' presentation in Chapter 1.

On Fridays some faculty members meet with Martha Rogers at New York University's Division of Nursing to discuss and revise the system. I recorded two such discussions in the fall of 1983 and extrapolated content from them, consisting primarily of Rogers' responses to ideas and questions from her colleagues. Each section represents a synthesis of the ideas expressed in both discussions.

PRECIS

The Science of Unitary Human Beings is a synthesis; as such it needs to be explored as a whole rather than piece by piece. For example, Rogers stated in one session that "theories derive from the system, not the building blocks." The Principles of Homeodynamics, taken together with the postulated correlates of patterning, demonstrate this synthesis.

ROGERS' POSTULATED CORRELATES OF PATTERNING IN UNITARY HUMAN BEINGS

Lower frequency	Higher frequency	Seem continuous
Longer rhythms	Shorter rhythms	Seem continuous
Slower motion	Faster motion	Seem continuous
Time drags	Time races	Timelessness
Sleeping	Waking	Beyond waking
Less diverse	More diverse	
Pragmatic	Imaginative	Visionary

Unitary human patterning, the distinguishing characteristic of an energy field perceived as a single wave, is creative and probabilistic. *Patterning* is a dynamic term, implying continuous change. The process of change is relative because each human–environmental field mutual process is unique. Change is also four-dimensional, negentropic, and nonlinear (these terms are presented in Chapter 3 for a comparison between Rogers' usage and that appearing in contemporary science), characterized by increasing diversity of field patterning.

Correlates of patterning emerge out of the human–environmental field mutual process. The list given here is not exhaustive; other correlatives need to be identified. However, those given provide direction for practice and research within this system. They encourage a "what-if" exploration of phenomena. For example, what if a hyperactive child is not displaying symptoms of a medical disorder but correlates of accelerated field patterning? He or she exhibits faster, more frequent motions; sleeps less; and perceives time as passing more quickly than do peers. Might field patterning, in terms of higher frequency light, color, and music, provide another approach to this child? Thus, observable behaviors are seen as manifestations of underlying field patterning, similar to a family therapist's interpretation of the behaviors of the "identified patient" as the symptoms of underlying problems in the total family system.

DISCUSSION

The discussion began with examples of frequently posed questions, such as "What would Martha Rogers say about nuclear war?" Those answers would go beyond the principles in the Science of Unitary Human Beings. At this point in the development of the system, discussants agreed that it is necessary to stay with what the principles say.

M. Rogers: You've hit on something that's a common thing. Everyone wants to know the pragmatics, whether it's nuclear holocaust or violence; all go to the negative, it seems. People have a difficult time seeing the difference in a hypothetical generalization or a unifying principle that doesn't deal with a specific, an "if–then" kind of thing, but rather as a guideline to set up probabilities, and that these characteristics or behaviors or events are really manifestations of the human–environmental field process. As such, what is the patterning involved? I tend to use the same old examples, but they're pretty good ones, like accelerating change, hypertension, and hyperactivity, in which pragmatics really emerge out of the principles.

Too often nurses fail to comprehend the scope of nursing, so they want to talk about it as something done in hospitals with sick people. That's only one setting. Our concern in the scope of nursing is people. That's nothing new; Nightingale certainly discussed it. I think when people get away from being narrowly oriented, they can better see the value of theories and principles in guiding whatever one calls nursing. Our concern is with people and the world they live in. Different settings are simply integral with the environment. People don't interact with a hospital; they interact with the total patterning of the environment.

Each energy field is unique to each human field; fields are continuously changing in the direction postulated, from lower to higher frequency wave patterns. *Patterning* is the operative word; the distinguishing characteristic of an energy field perceived as a single wave.

Respondent: That makes a lot of sense. You know how you can walk through the door going home after work and know what kind of an evening you're going to have—this wave just hits you in the face. A nurse in practice can walk onto a unit and just know it's going to be one of those days. You really do pick up the environment as a single phenomenon. It's later that you go back and try to pick out particular things, but the perception is a unified one.

M. Rogers: We're dealing with an individual whole. The conceptual system is a synthesis; in a synthesis there are no more building blocks, and we don't go in to test the building blocks or predict behaviors on the basis of them. Rather, it's the total configuration.

Respondent: That's a problem I have with the definition, "perceived as a single wave." This seems to suggest that this totality is somehow being condensed into a part. Is this what our three-dimensional perception can perceive?

M. Rogers: It's not a condensation but a synthesis . . . the example of a radio wave . . . coming out are multiple manifestations of the patterning rather than multiple frequencies. What one brings in is on a single frequency. If one thinks of human and environmental fields as a pattern, we perceive the totality of a pattern—that's a field manifestation, and it is on a single frequency, not a collection of frequencies. Here there are not parts; patterning transcends.

CORRELATES OF PATTERNING

M. Rogers: Originally those were correlates of human development. Well, that didn't fit, because development implies certain kinds of linearity. These are now talked about as correlates of patterning; it's nonlinear change. Nonrepeating rhythmicities are similarities, never the same, but they can give us clues.

In *An Introduction to the Theoretical Basis of Nursing* (1970), I talked about unidirectionality. What I said didn't transmit what I thought. As generally used, it's linear, whereas what I mean is that patterning is always changing in the direction of innovation and growing diversity. It's probabilistic, so that one can't be sure of exact changes. It deals with the relative nature of change.

Chronological age is not a useful tool for predicting in this system. Correlates are just manifestations that are integral with the growing diversity of pattern that I refer to as higher frequency.

If, as I postulate, change is continuous and in the direction of increasing diversity of patterning, no matter what's happening in this increasing diversity of pattern, there are similarities but never the same [pattern repeated]. I think this may be tied to our capacity to perceive; we're caught in temporality. If we consider the present not as a point in time but plus or minus 25,000 years, it is similarities in patterning that are nonrepetitive, always more diverse, but providing clues. Correlates are manifestations of field. Correlates aren't four-dimensional per se; it's the total system, not any part of the system. A four-dimensional field will manifest sleeping as much as beyond waking. It doesn't mean these are four-dimensional and these are not (some correlates as opposed to others).

Respondent: But all of these things can be manifested in energy fields; it's not like, if you have one, you don't have the others.

M. Rogers: Oh, no. And we've been thinking about adding to the list to get more correlates. These continue to provide operational phenomena that can be helpful in research. I was using this list in class 20 years ago; now it's well documented that people sleep less at every age than they did 30 or 40 years ago. There are findings that support the postulated direction of change. Rhythms have picked up. But as I said, these are manifestations of patterning, of this growing diversity.

FOUR-DIMENSIONALITY

M. Rogers: When quantum theory came in, we talked about acausality, not "this came before that" and "A before B." I do think the whole question of temporality is an exceedingly difficult one. . . . It's well dug into our thinking. I've defined *four-dimensionality* as "without spatial or temporal attributes." I think that's a good definition, but trying to explain it is something else again.

The use of Therapeutic Touch as an intervention modality requires some kind of a perception of four-dimensionality, whether they (Therapeutic Touch practitioners) can spell it out or not. This is a manifestation of this conceptual system.

We're not evolving into four-dimensionality from three-dimensionality . . . four-dimensionality has no meaning at all except within the total system. The correlates are manifestations of pattern; these are observable phenomena that don't derive from the field or four-dimensionality. They derive from the totality of the system.

ACCELERATING CHANGE; DIVERSITY OF PATTERNING

M. Rogers: The relative nature of change is manifesting itself in greater diversity, and the range of differences is vastly greater than it's ever been. Because four-dimensionality is without temporal or spatial attributes . . . moving from the present as a point in time and trying to avoid linearity, the relative nature of change becomes very important. Even relativity, when it began to move away into nonlinear constructs, was still a three-dimensional perception for most people. Some places I've seen this referred to as the "infinite now," which I think makes more sense.

What I believe is important is accepting people as they are and helping them achieve their own potentials instead of the hierarchical "good–better–best" perspective. Continuous change is going to take place anyway. It's the nature of the pattern that becomes important.

The only thing is the pattern, and pattern not only comes through as a single wave but we get into diversity of patterning, and it's diversity of patterning that we're talking about with "relative." The pattern of my environmental field is different from each one of yours.

Everything is always unique. [There may be] marked similarity, but the same kind of argument I would use in relation to fingerprints, voiceprints . . . twinning—even those who are most alike still are not identical, except to gross observation.

There seems to be an increase of so-called "paranormal" phenomena, which I propose are more and more becoming so-called "normal." This would tie itself into growing diversity. The more diverse pattern manifests these kinds of characteristics in ways that the less diverse did not . . . a pattern that manifests phenomena currently labeled "paranormal." All that "paranormal" means is something we haven't accepted traditionally as normal.

Even the little bit we've seen in relation to astronauts, this observable physical body does change in size, shape, the works. We do know that life forms transcend themselves in the direction of greater diversity. We are moving toward whole different patterns; moon villages and space towns are going to be a reality before the year 2000.

The problem I got into with the term "development" is it's been used to signify physical, emotional, or social development, a form of segmentation and adding up the parts. I think it's difficult to take terms with heavily stereotyped meanings and use them to signify something else. So while I think that in a global sense this human field manifests changes that can be labeled development, it would not be the same thing as in the traditional ways, traditional meanings of development. Therefore, I think it's better not to use the term. *Patterning* does say what we are talking about and also leaves the door open for innovative change that will begin to explain some of the manifestations we've seen in this period of acceleration.

FIELD

M. Rogers: Fields are infinite; there can be millions of fields. Cell biologists talk about cellular fields, but the two fields I talk about are human and environmental. Since fields are infinite, and these fields are integral with one another, inseparable and different only by virtue of patterning, there are no other fields when one is dealing with these two. The concept "field" is a unifying concept. Energy is a dynamic concept, so we have two integral fields that are dynamic unity.

People don't differentiate between this physical being and a human field. When you try to illustrate, they say you have a field around you. There is no such thing as a field around; the person is a field, he doesn't have one. [In death for example,] the patterning continues in frequencies that are outside the traditional. The field is perceived in certain kinds of patterning. If we're talking about the human being, we're talking about a field, not a physical body. The fact that it happens to be perceived in certain kinds of patterning [doesn't mean that's what it is]. Our capacity to perceive is very, very limited. We can see the seeds in the apple, but can we see the apple in the seed? You have to think of a nonspatial, nontemporal, infinite energy field that you perceive according to patterning . . . an energy field is dynamic. An energy field is motion . . . in the physical world movement is point-to-point, but in the nonlinear world, it's not.

Nobody's ever seen a field. [Some have] seen something they call manifestations. People refer to the aura, but I would say that's no more the field than saying somebody has a field around them. All they're doing is seeing something that happens to fall within a visible range for some people. Some people do perceive in higher and lower frequency wave patterns, this in a visible range that is broader than the one we've counted as average. But that's not the field; it's a manifestation of the field. [For example] Kirlian photography* brings into view aspects of field that other ways of looking didn't.

We need to change our way of dealing with events and to use a descriptive approach. . . . I think what we need to do in nursing is get away from categorical entities and use descriptive approaches to identify what it is you're going to study. If anybody else wants to use such categories, and certainly we need to communicate with people in other fields, it has to be handled almost like teaching a foreign language. In terms of nursing, certainly description is reputedly a valid aid in any developing science. I think another resource in terms of research that we haven't used very much yet is phenomenology. Description and phenomenology both provide further ways of trying to look at these things.

Editor's Note
Perhaps it is becoming clear that there are no "answers," in the sense of last words or final resolutions, within this system. The world view underlying the Science of Unitary Human Beings, one of total openness and continuous change, fosters ongoing inquiry.

---

* A means of capturing an image of what is reported to be the aura of energy emanating from living things.

3

Contemporary Science and Nursing: Parallels with Rogers

Violet M. Malinski

In contemporary thought new world views are emerging that offer a different way of looking at people and the world. Inherent in such views are the primacy of the human–environment interaction process and a belief in the underlying unity of life. In nursing, for example, Rogers maintains that the uniqueness of the nursing profession arises from its focus on human beings and their world, which she sees as a logical step to the development of a conceptual system for nursing that offers a view of people and their environments as integral wholes evolving together via a continuous, mutual process of interaction.[16]

Similar ideas, some of which are novel while others can be traced back over the ages, are emerging in other fields and seem to be converging into a world view with which Rogers shares certain parallels. Contributing to this view, for example, are the ideas of theoretical physicists Capra (the interconnectedness of the universe, mass as dynamic energy patterning, probability rather than linear cause-effect) and Bohm (holonomy or undivided wholeness, acausal correlations), neuroscientist Pribram (holographic model of the brain), chemist Prigogine (increasing order and complexity in open systems), biologist Sheldrake (hypothesis of causative formation), anthropologist Bateson (the pattern that connects, the unity of thought and evolution), and futurist–economist Henderson (solar politics).[1, 2, 5–7, 9–14, 17, 18]

With this proliferation of ideas, it is possible that we are building toward a critical mass similar to Watson's "hundredth-monkey phenomenon," a process whereby "new" knowledge becomes common knowledge once assimilated by a sufficient core of group members.[19] In Watson's example, the first monkey to think of washing grit off sweet potatoes taught others by example until the one hundredth monkey learned to wash sweet potatoes. At that point, as though some threshold had been crossed, all the monkeys on that and neighboring islands were soon washing sweet potatoes; somehow this behavior had become part of the repertoire of all the monkeys in the area. Perhaps a similar process is at work behind a gradual shifting of world views.

THE IMPORTANCE OF WORLD VIEWS

World views condition perceptions, while the values associated with them reflect dominant belief systems. The perception of "reality" varies when we see the whole as a collection of independent parts versus as a unitary, coherent entity. According to Bohm, the prevailing or traditional world view favors a fragmented self–world perception, following the Cartesian tradition of mind–body duality.[2] Descartes based his view of nature on the distinction between mind and matter; objective description became the scientific ideal. Another characteristic of the traditional world view is the static, mechanistic picture of human and universe developed in Newtonian or classical physics. Newton viewed the universe as a world-machine, set in motion at the creation, which will eventually run out of energy and cease to function. The human body, within this framework, is also perceived as a reacting machine possessing finite energy resources.

In medicine this view has resulted in the search for the defective part. Fix it or replace it with an artificial or transplanted one, and the body will function properly again. Isolate the microbe and you will eradicate the disease. Although this approach often produces the desired results, its explanations and range of activities are limited. Perhaps one of the major factors behind the current crisis in medical care is the adherence to a reductionistic, mechanistic philosophy.

In contrast to medicine, nursing has traditionally espoused a holistic or "total-person" view, although this has been operationalized very often as a way of looking at parts and trying to build up to the whole. As a nurse one of the first things I learned was the importance of context, defined as the whole situation, background, or that which is relevant to a person or event.[20] This meant working with the person in the context of family, community, cultural group. I also learned that a strict cause–effect model had limited applicability; 10 people exposed to the same microbe would not necessarily each catch the disease. There was another element to be considered: the interaction between person and environment. I was not conscious, however, of having a world view in which these were integral factors. Throughout my educational experiences Rogers was the first to put forth a coherent world view and distinguish it from what she saw as the prevailing world view.[15]

CONTRASTING PREVAILING VIEWS VERSUS ROGERS' VIEW OF PEOPLE

Prevailing View	Rogers' View
Cell theory	Field theory
Entropic universe	Negentropic universe
Man: three-dimensional	Human being: four-dimensional

Prevailing View	Rogers' View
Man: homeostatic	Human being: homeodynamic
Man–environment: dichotomous	Human being–environment: integral
Man: summation of parts	Human being: unitary
Causation: single and multiple	Continuous mutual process
Adaptation	Continuous mutual process
Closed systems: feedback	Open systems: probability, innovation
Dynamic equilibrium	Innovative growing complexity
Waking: man's basic state	Waking: an evolutionary emergent
Spatialization of time	Dynamization of space
Present: point in time	Present: multidimensional
Being	Becoming

What is the essence of a world view emerging today, and what does it have in common with Rogers' view identified here?

WORLD VIEWS EMERGING IN CONTEMPORARY THOUGHT

The main concepts developed by twentieth-century physics are those of relativity and the quantum principle.[21] Relativity has demonstrated that "mutability is the law of nature,"[21] supplanting the absolutes of time and space in Newtonian physics. Quantum theory disclosed the basic oneness of a universe characterized by patterns of energy rather than by bounded substance; by tendencies–probabilities to exist, to behave, to occur, rather than linear cause–effect—a dynamic web of relationships that includes both observer and observed.[7] Thus the scientific ideal of the objective observer has been called into question, with recognition given to the dynamics of the interplay between observer and observed as a unitary process.[21]

The classical view of the world as a collection of distinct yet interacting parts, divisible into particles and fields, has yielded to a new order in quantum theory, "the order of undivided wholeness," characterized by acausal correlations.[2] According to Capra, quantum theory has demonstrated that the boundaries used to separate and contain matter are artifacts; "the whole universe appears as a dynamic web of inseparable energy patterns."[7] The idea of mass as substance has been modified to mass as a dynamic pattern of energy.[7] Matter, having both particle and wave aspects, is bounded within a small volume yet, at the same time, spread over space, two seemingly contradictory statements. A particle can be understood only as a manifestation of an interaction process, not "an isolated entity, but . . . an integrated part of the whole."[7]

By transcending the Cartesian duality and the classical ideal of the objective observer, modern physics has also challenged the value-neutral position of science.[6] Because the patterns that scientists observe in nature are intimately bound with the patterns of their minds, the results obtained and the technologies derived will be connected to their thoughts and values. The crises that we encounter today arise from our persistence in trying to apply concepts from the traditional world view when reality can no longer be comprehended within its terms.[6]

Bateson and Henderson argued in a similar vein, charging that the premises arising out of the traditional world view have led to greed, war, overgrowth, and pollution.[1, 9] According to Henderson, we are in transition from a fossil-fuel age, characterized by a dependence on stored capital (oil, coal), paternalism, oppression, manipulative technologies designed to control, and a reductionist philosophy, to a Solar Age where we shall have to rely on daily income from the sun and regain our ecological awareness and appreciation for interrelationships rather than dominance and control.

The Cartesian mind–body duality gives rise to the demarcating of boundaries, a process of compartmentalization. According to Bateson, however, boundaries, if they exist at all, are not spatial entities, but more like Venn diagrams or "the bubbles that come out of the mouths of the characters in comic strips,"[1] artifacts created for our convenience. He suggested that it is time to set aside Cartesian duality in favor of the recognition that the two systems of thought and evolution form one integrated whole. The individual's "knowing" is but a small slice of a wider knowledge that knits the entire biosphere. What become important, then, are relationships, not objects, patterns that evolve through time and the context that elucidates them.

Relativity and quantum theories imply undivided wholeness, whereby analysis of the parts becomes irrelevant.[2] In shifting our focus from the parts that form the whole to the whole as a fundamental reality that is more than and different from the sum of its parts, patterning is the key to understanding.

For Bohm, holonomy is the law of the whole.[2] He has proposed a holonomic model of the universe according to which there is a single, unbroken flow of existence that contains both consciousness and external reality.[2] As indicated by use of the word *flow,* Bohm conceives of this as a dynamic process, one of movement, the enfolding and unfolding of holomovement, and it occurs in multidimensional reality, transcending the limitations of three-dimensional reality. The intrinsic order in this cosmic web of relations is called the *implicate* or *enfolded* order. As a matrix of inseparable connections among all things, it forms the ground of the holomovement. It is infinite, without boundaries. This is the wave or frequency domain. The implicate is made explicit by the process of unfolding or holomovement. What we consider reality is actually a projection or manifestation of this underlying totality. Each individual is such a projection and, therefore, is in total contact with the implicate order, where everything is present at once. This conceptualization of implicate order can help us understand such phenomena as intuition, empathy, healing across distances, and precognition.

Bohm uses the hologram as an aid to understanding "undivided wholeness," pointing out that the word is derived from the Greek *holo* (whole) and *gram* (to write), an instrument that "writes the whole."[2] In holography, coherent light (single frequency) from a laser passes through a half-silvered mirror and is split so that part of the beam shines on a photographic plate while the other half is reflected off the object to be reconstructed. When the reflected light reaches the photographic plate, it "interferes" with the light already shining on the plate, thus setting up an interference pattern that is recorded on the plate. Once a beam of light is shown on this plate, the original object is reconstructed in three-dimensional space as though it were physically there. The form and structure of the object have been enfolded onto the photographic plate. Furthermore, because this information has been distributed across the plate in the form of an interference *pattern,* light shown through any part of the plate can be used to reconstitute or unfold the whole [image]; the whole is contained in the part.

Pribram compared this distributive property of the hologram to that of the brain, postulating that cerebral excitation results in the formation of something analogous to a hologram in the brain.[10-12] One of the keys in Pribram's development of his holographic proposal was the work of Karl Lashley, who speculated that sensory input to the cortex generates waves of activity that interact to produce interference patterns.[11] Such a distribution of information across the brain could account for the apparent distribution of memory throughout the brain. For example, brain lesions cannot be linked to the disappearance of specific memories.

Holography demonstrates the reciprocal relationship between the frequency (lightwave) domain and the image–object domain.[10] The frequency domain is characteristic of brain processing; it is also what Bohm calls the *implicate order.* The images that the brain constructs to fit our three-dimensional perception are emergents or manifestations, the implicate made explicit. Pribram speculated that if the brain and physical universe do share in an implicate holographic order, each represents the other. The part represents the whole [universe] while the universe "implies" the part.[12]

The dynamic nature of dissipative structures may be the bridge linking the ideas of Bohm and Pribram to those of Prigogine, who discusses the physics of being and the physics of becoming.[13, 14] The former deals with reversible phenomena, while the latter explores irreversible ones as described by the second law of thermodynamics. In the nonequilibrium (the flow of matter and energy) world in which we live, the second law—that everything is running down or increasing in entropy—does not hold true for some open systems, dissipative structures, or dynamic states, which dissipate entropy into the environment with which they interact and thus "run up" or increase in complexity. Under nonequilibrium conditions, the very interaction of a system with the environment "may become in this way the starting point for the formation of new dynamic states of matter—dissipative structures."[14] Irreversibility is the source of order and embraces the concept of time, which, in open systems, is irreversible. Because we tend to perceive reality as embedded in a flowing stream of time, time and reality are related.[14] Within the arrow of time, "The past is included, but the future remains uncertain."[14] We can only deal with probabilities, nonlinear forces in the process of emergence.

Sheldrake[17, 18] has put forth the hypothesis of formative causation, an evolutionary view of reality in which morphogenetic fields serve as archetypes by which to shape forms and transmit information. This process is a reciprocal one; the field affects and is affected by the organism. The field is nonlocal, thus acting outside of time and space by a process called *morphic resonance.* A system has a characteristic pattern of vibration and internal rhythms; it "becomes *present* to a subsequent system with a similar form. . . ."[17] For example, chemists often have difficulty when first trying to crystallize new chemical compounds, yet the substances crystallize more readily as time goes on. The usual explanation has been that fragments of the earlier crystals "seed" the newer compounds. According to Sheldrake's hypothesis of formative causation, crystallization should occur more readily as the increasing numbers of compounds crystallized contribute to the morphogenetic field via morphic resonance,[17] perhaps another way to look at Watson's hundredth-monkey phenomenon.[19]

Because Sheldrake's hypothesis encompasses physical form and habitual patterns of behavior, essentially repetitive events, he has left open the question of creativity. He explored it in a discussion of morphogenetic fields and the implicate order with Bohm, who suggested that the field could be viewed as a set of potentialities interacting with past history and creativity in the actualization of one potential over another.[3] This relationship of past to future brings in time, which Bohm conceptualizes as moments of potentialities and actualities, with the actuality of the previous moment connected to the potentiality of the next—"introjection . . . of the actuality of the past into that field from which the present is going to be projected."[3] Sheldrake sees evolution as a creative process and speculated that it "could be seen as a successive development of more complex and higher level wholes, through previously separate things being connected together."[3] Given the idea of an evolutionary universe, the notion that timeless laws govern the natural world ceases to make sense;[8] hence Prigogine's distinction between phenomena governed by the second law of thermodynamics and those that are not.

Although embedded within different theoretical bases, Rogers' model interfaces with the emerging world views just described. This is especially the case in the recognition of the wave nature of life and the unitary process of the human–environment interaction. Major differences also exist, as they do among all the authors discussed. As might be expected, given the opening distinction between traditional and emerging world views, each is controversial, reflecting the inherent differences in outlook between those espousing alternative world views.

ROGERS' SCIENCE OF UNITARY HUMAN BEINGS

As noted earlier, Rogers contrasts the world view underlying her model with what she identified as the prevailing view. Selected aspects will be presented in this section and compared to ideas discussed in the preceding section.

Field; Synergism (Whole Is More Than the Sum of the Parts)

Both Rogers and Capra identify "field" as the fundamental, unifying concept; both see fields as having no boundaries. For Capra, fields link particles and the space surrounding them, blurring the distinction between matter and empty space characteristic of Newtonian physics.[7] Rogers defines both unitary human beings and environment as four-dimensional, irreducible energy fields characterized by patterning, the perception of the field as a single wave. What is accessible to three-dimensional perception is an index of the underlying four-dimensional process, although human and environment do not have dual wave–particle aspects in Rogers' view but are four-dimensional energy fields coextensive with the universe.

Discussing field from the theoretical physicist's stance, Capra points out that relativity theory tells us that mass is a form of energy.[7] Although the definition of *field* varies between Rogers and Capra, the idea that underlying everything is energy patterning seems consistent. Bohm, on the other hand, uses field (and particles) as an abstraction to facilitate comprehension of a universe that cannot be subdivided into any interacting parts.[2] Rogers would agree with this last statement, viewing the unitary human being and the environment as irreducible energy fields coextensive with the universe. As opposed to the concept of field in physics, Rogers is not talking about it in the sense of gravitational or electromagnetic fields. Nor is she talking about the morphogenetic or M-field, as Sheldrake does. His seems a more particulate idea than those espoused by the other three, focusing specifically on the repetition of past forms.

Each person discussed earlier varies in the interpretation of the whole as more than and different from the sum of the parts or as an extrapolation from the parts. For example, Rogers, Bohm, and Capra tend to look at wholes as synergistic, whereas Bateson saw parts as useful in describing the whole. Pribram, by virtue of his focus on the brain and neurological functioning, presents a particulate approach in contrast to Rogers. Her model does not deal with the functioning of any particular organ or system, but interprets all behaviors as an index to the whole.

Human Being–Environment: Complementary

Each of the authors discussed espouses a complementary view of our relationship with our world, as opposed to perceiving the person and the environment as dichotomous, with humanity dominating and controlling nature, for example. Rogers' principle of integrality identifies the unitary interaction of human and environment. The essential, underlying unity of all things comes across strongly in the writings of Capra, Bohm, Prigogine, Bateson, and Henderson, but is also seen in Sheldrake's view of the reciprocal relationship between field and organism and Pribram's assertion that each organism in some way represents the universe, and vice versa.

Negentropic Universe; Open Systems: Probability, Innovation; Innovative Growing Complexity; Becoming

Prigogine's work seems to present the clearest parallels to Rogers' view. As noted earlier, he deals with the "physics of becoming" as contrasted to the "physics of being" and has demonstrated through chemical reactions that change in open systems is probabilistic and in the direction of increasing complexity. Rather than an entropic universe, a static one that is evolving from order to disorder, we live in a negentropic universe characterized by increasing order and complexity whose evolution is irreversible.

Rogers' principle of helicy shows the nature and direction of change (innovative, nonrepeating, probabilistic) while the principle of resonancy specifies its modality—wave patterning from lower to higher frequencies. She postulates change as a process of emergence, where what emerges via the dynamic patterning of the field is always innovative and unpredictable rather than a manifestation of what has always been there and not directly accessible to consciousness.

Where Sheldrake has focused more on repetition of past forms, Bohm allows for difference and innovation in the sense that every new moment can be unrelated to the previous one and so is totally creative.[5] Where Bohm seems to differ from Rogers is in his acceptance of modified repetition. To paraphrase Bohm, a form emerges from the whole (the implicate order) creatively; influences or is injected back into the whole, where it resonates with similar forms; and is then reprojected from the implicate order; again, the implicate made explicate.[5]

Present: Multidimensional; Four-Dimensionality

Within Rogers' model time does not exist in the linear sense of movement from the past through the present toward the future. Rather, she uses the term "relative present" to denote four-dimensional field differences in the experience of time; what is "present" for one may not be for another (see Chapter 2).

In classical or Newtonian physics, space and time were perceived as separate and absolute, with time flowing independent of the material world, whereas modern physics has demonstrated that time and space are connected and interpenetrated in a four-dimensional continuum where interactions can extend in any direction.[7] This is a dynamic view in which time and change are seen as essential. It allows for the idea of higher states of consciousness; for example, the timeless present of the mystics, rather than a linear succession of moments.[7] Although Capra discusses four-dimensionality in relation to time, Rogers' view of four-dimensionality is not the same as that in physics; she is referring to a domain that is both nonlinear and *without* attributes of space and time.

Bohm conceives time as a projection of multidimensional reality, not as an absolute, linear flow but as multidimensional orders of sequences of moments.[2] Time is unfolded from the implicate order. Creativity again comes into play, for no one sequence of moments is totally derivable from that which preceded it. As in Rogers' view, what is present for one person may not be for another.

SUMMARY

Although conceptual differences exist, a number of ideas emerging in contemporary thought appear consistent with those Rogers has proposed over the years; for example:

- Human and environment are unified wholes more than and different from the sum of their parts

• Human and environment are energy fields engaged in mutual, simultaneous interaction evolving in the direction of increasing complexity and diversity of patterning
• They are coextensive with the universe
• Time and space are relative, providing, for example, a base within which to view paranormal phenomena

The following chapter examines the practice implications of Rogers' model. Subsequent chapters present research formulated within the model, reintroducing some of the ideas discussed earlier.

REFERENCES

1. Bateson G: Mind and Nature, a Necessary Unity. New York, Bantam Books, 1979
2. Bohm D: Wholeness and the Implicate Order. Boston, Routledge & Kegan Paul, 1980
3. Bohm D, Sheldrake R: Morphogenetic fields and the implicate order. ReVision 5:41–48, 1982
4. Bohm D, Weber R: The enfolding–unfolding universe, a conversation with David Bohm. ReVision 1:24–51, 1978
5. Bohm D, Weber R: Nature as creativity. ReVision 5:35–40, 1982
6. Capra F: The Turning Point; Science, Society, and the Rising Culture. New York, Simon & Schuster, 1982
7. Capra F: The Tao of Physics, 2nd ed. New York, Bantam Books, 1983
8. Conversations between Rupert Sheldrake, Renee Weber, David Bohm, Introduction. ReVision 5:23–26, 1982
9. Henderson H: The Politics of the Solar Age, Alternatives to Economics. New York, Anchor Press/Doubleday, 1981
10. Pribram K: What the fuss is all about. ReVision 1:14–18, 1978
11. Pribram K: The role of analogy in transcending limits in the brain sciences. Daedalus 109:19–38, 1980
12. Pribram K: Behaviorism, phenomenology, and holism in psychology: A scientific analysis. In Valle RS, von Eckartsberg R (eds): The Metaphors of Consciousness. New York, Plenum Press, 1981, pp 141–151
13. Prigogine I: From Being to Becoming, Time and Complexity in the Physical Sciences. San Francisco, W. H. Freeman & Company, 1980
14. Prigogine I, Stengers I: Order Out of Chaos, Man's New Dialogue with Nature. New York, Bantam Books, 1984
15. Rogers ME: Contrasting prevailing view versus Rogers' view of people. Class handout, The Science of Man. New York University Division of Nursing, Fall, 1976
16. Rogers ME: Science of unitary human beings: A paradigm for nursing, 1983 (unpublished)
17. Sheldrake R: A New Science of Life, the Hypothesis of Formative Causation. Los Angeles, J. P. Tarcher, 1981
18. Sheldrake R, Weber R: Morphogenetic fields: Nature's habits. ReVision 5:27–34, 1982
19. Watson L: Lifetide, the Biology of the Unconscious. New York, Bantam Books, 1979
20. Webster's New World Dictionary, 2nd ed. New York, Simon & Schuster, 1980
21. Wheeler JA: From relativity to mutability. In Mehra J (ed): The physicist's conception of nature. Boston, D. Reidel, 1973, pp 202–247

4

Nursing Practice within the Science of Unitary Human Beings

Violet M. Malinski

When people read Rogers' model for the first time, many question its relevance for practice. Although this is an important question, I would like to pose a slightly different one. After exploring the Science of Unitary Human Beings, how has my world view changed and with it the way I practice nursing?

The previous chapter explored the implications of a world view, comparing and contrasting Rogers' ideas with some of those appearing in other fields. In this chapter, a framework for practice and trends derived from the model are discussed.

THE FRAMEWORK FOR NURSING PRACTICE

World views condition perceptions, while values reflect dominant belief systems. As Einstein said, the theory determines what we can observe. The importance of world views was explored in Chapter 3 and sets the stage for this discussion, because our beliefs and values determine what we can accept as options for practice within the Science of Unitary Human Beings. As scientists cannot claim to be value-neutral (see Chapter 3), neither can health care providers. Belief that something will work on the part of both client and provider is connected with success or failure.

If we accept that the person is an energy field, then it is easy to explore as treatment modalities Therapeutic Touch, meditation, or music. If we accept the

A version of this chapter was presented at the First National Rogerian Conference, New York University, June 24–26, 1983.

integral connectedness of person and environment, then the idea that the healing milieu is as important as the treatment modality does not seem strange. Nor does the idea that the belief about a treatment modality and the attitude of the health care provider toward the client (desire to help, annoyance, labeling the person as noncompliant) are integral to the field interaction seem strange. The placebo effect has been well documented.

Inherent in the conception of the person as an energy field is the idea that we extend beyond our skins. Because fields are defined as coextensive with the universe, thus without boundaries, everything is interconnected through energy patterning. The underlying patterning of the human field, for example, is manifested in what we can observe most directly, the physical body and behaviors of a person. Because everything is interrelated, there are correlations but no one cause. Fields are irreducible wholes. Wholeness implies concern with the totality of the person in interaction with the environment.

Therapeutic Touch* provides a useful illustration for understanding wholeness. Pioneered by Krieger, Therapeutic Touch is a conscious, intentional act performed in the service of healing.[10, 11] From her readings of Eastern literature, Krieger learned about a life energy called *prana*. Healthy people have it in abundance; sick people do not have enough. Krieger's conception of Therapeutic Touch is rooted in the assumption that the human being is an open system, thus interacting with the environment and sensitive to wave phenomena such as energy. She sees the healer as a healthy person with an abundance of prana who could channel this energy flow for the benefit of the healee based on a strong commitment or intention to help the ill person. This channeling of energy would re-establish the healee's own energy flow, restoring communication between human and environmental fields, enabling the healee to mobilize his or her own innate healing forces.[11] Krieger believes that Therapeutic Touch, like self-healing, is a natural potential existing in people that can be activated provided they are motivated to help others and are able to confront themselves honestly in answering why they want to be healers.[11]

A nurse using Therapeutic Touch works with the person as a whole.[13] If someone has abdominal cramps, the nurse does not focus immediately on the abdomen but works on the total energy field, moving from head to feet, assessing and unruffling† the field, balancing the flow of energy.[9] The focus is on the whole person, not on the area of the body where the person experiences discomfort. Symptoms would be explored within the context of the total process. Consonant with the concept of energy fields, it is not necessary to touch the person physically throughout this process, although the nurse may do so.[16]

Given that people and environment are integral, that all is related within a dynamic flow of energy patterning, life and health‡ are seen as processes rather

---

* Therapeutic Touch is not derived from Rogers' system, but parallels can be drawn between ideas in both views.

† The phase of Therapeutic Touch in which the healer facilitates the movement of congested energy.

‡ Rogers does not discuss health, seeing this as a value term.[21] The author's perspective is offered as a focus for discussion.

than as fixed points denoting the ends of continua, e.g, Health————Illness, Life————Death. Instead, living–dying is a rhythmic process. Rogers speculates that the continuity of field patterning continues after death.[20] We cannot cure someone who is dying, but we can assist that person and family toward a healthy death.[6]

From the perspective of this model, we are coming to understand that health, an index of field patterning, is interaction evolving from the continuous mutual process of human and environmental fields. It is a lived experience in which nurses can participate as facilitators and educators, as advocates, assessors, planners, coordinators, and as collaborators in therapeutic relationships with clients, helping them become attuned to their own unique rhythms and patterning.

Individuals have their own unique ways of being and their own creative potentials but are grounded in and evolve from the whole. Behaviors that are manifested by the human field are not viewed as end states to diagnose and treat but as manifestations of the underlying process, or patterning. In communication theory it is said that one cannot *not* communicate. Refusing to communicate is a communication in itself, whether one of anger, hurt, or another emotion. We communicate with gestures, expressions, and body positions in addition to words. In the same way, we can never *not* interact. The energy field is always open, even if the manifestation is labeled "catatonic schizophrenic" or "comatose." The key is interaction, energy patterns flowing through energy patterns.

We can explore illness and disease in terms of the meanings they hold for the persons involved and their intrinsic potentials for growth, although it is important that this idea not be translated into a "blaming-the-victim" stance in which some value judgement is made about the quality of a person's interactions with others or lifestyle. The perspective of a Comanche medicine man comes to mind. He believed that we have a free choice in terms of health and illness, that sickness is an experience chosen to facilitate learning, and that we have the capacity to heal ourselves. He used himself as an example, explaining that he had had rheumatoid arthritis as a child and was also rigid in his beliefs. As he learned to become more flexible in his thinking, his body became more flexible. In Rogers' terms, we can participate knowingly to activate some potentials over others; we have options.

Within the Science of Unitary Human Beings, both nurse and client participate in the mobilization of health potentials. Krieger has learned from her practice of Therapeutic Touch that it is the healee who heals her- or himself.[10] Clients have self-knowledge to share; they need to become attuned to their own rhythms, not disconnected from them.

The ability to mobilize health potential may be connected to accepting that nothing is static and fixed for all time, as in the classical view of the body and universe in Newtonian physics, but temporary, dynamic, and continuously changing (see Chapter 3). Change is not only possible; it is the "norm." Departing from a linear, cause–effect view of the world, we come to probabilistic outcomes. In some cancers, a diagnosis does not necessarily mean death. Death, a possible outcome, may be the probable one if the person so diagnosed accepts this meaning as the only or inevitable one.

The images people hold of themselves are important to their ability to mobilize self-healing potential.[1, 12, 22] Those who use imagery with cancer patients, for example, have found a correlation between strength of the image and the person's progress.

Nursing's concern for unitary human beings incorporates other nurses and health care providers as well as ourselves as we recognize that attitudes, intentions, and feelings toward those with whom we work are an integral part of an interaction process. We can learn how to take better care of ourselves and contribute to healthy, supportive environments in which our creativity flourishes. Perhaps the main question to pose as we explore practice in Rogers' Science of Unitary Human Beings is: What kind of role models are we becoming in the process?

PRACTICE TRENDS

1. Empowering both nurse and client: Women and nurses, as groups with considerable overlap between them, have had difficulty with the concept of power in the traditional usage of power over, or power to use against, others. Rich identified power as energy looking for an object into which to pour itself, perhaps as flowing between people.[19] Starhawk equated "power over" with the power of annihilation, while "power within" arises from the understanding that everything is connected; all is relationship.[23] Rather than viewing power dualistically—those who have versus those who do not—empowerment seems appropriate within Rogers' model.

Empowerment of clients means recognizing them as equal partners in the health care system and sharing knowledge and skills with them, enabling clients to exercise their autonomy in deciding which options to choose. Rather than labeling them resistant, nurses need to acknowledge that some clients may not be able or willing to participate and be available to them when they are ready to do so. It is possible that behavior typically labeled "resistant" or "noncompliant" is actually healthy behavior on the part of the client. As a friend stated following a lengthy hospitalization and cancer therapy regime, he finally figured out that if he was going to live and make progress, he had to get out of the hospital and away from the doctors and their treatments. It became quite clear that if he did not, he was going to die. Cousins' *Anatomy of an Illness* provides a clear illustration of the potential role to be played by the patient in his or her own care, enhancing body chemistry by the use of a range of positive emotions, including laughter.[4]

Nursing, a Social Policy Statement, recognized that people have responsibility for their own health and for developing those potentials for achieving it.[2] Rather than trying to exercise any power of authority over clients and trying to make them comply with what health care providers want, nurses need to provide health teaching and other tools that enable clients to choose knowledgeably.

2. Accepting diversity as the norm: This means not only respect for differences but a genuine appreciation for diversity. The environment is different for each human; patterning is unique to the human field. For example, the recognition that hyperactive children may be children of high frequency patterning (see Chapter 10) challenges nurses to search for alternate strategies, such as multistimuli learning centers using light, color, and music; incorporation of creative imaging and meditation; music and movement; all of which can be done in homes, schools, and treatment centers.[15]

There is a growing recognition that health itself is a relative term. (As noted earlier, Rogers has chosen not to use the term ''health'' because of the value connotations it carries.) The definitions of health and health problems vary among cultural groups. Many Navajo, for example, have congenital hip dislocations, which they do not regard as a problem because the dislocation does not interfere with daily life. What does interfere and thus constitute a problem is the treatment, a surgically fused hip, which prevents the Navajo from sitting cross-legged on the floor of the hogan with friends and riding a horse to round up the sheep.

Within the theory of accelerating change, we expect to see changing norms. Diversity becomes the norm, fostering respect for persons.

3. Becoming attuned to patterning: This is manifested in such rhythmic correlates as sleep and perception of time passing, and in feelings for certain colors and music. Nurses can assist clients to become aware of their own rhythms and to make choices among a range of options congruent with their perceptions of well-being, from structuring environments using light and color to meditation, including Therapeutic Touch as a healing meditation.[10] In order to do this, we nurses have the right as well as the responsibility to do the same for ourselves. Our rhythms are equally important.

4. Recognizing and using wave modalities such as light, color, music, and movement as integral to the patterning process and thus to health and healing: Color and music, for example, have been used in healing rituals since ancient times. Light has a history of therapeutic applications from bilirubin to cancer therapies and is an important consideration in human health.[24]

Light and other wave forms have not been fully integrated into nursing practice yet. Their use forms the basis of various treatment approaches and assists in structuring environments, whether homes, schools, or institutional settings, to promote optimal well-being. Music and movement, as manifestations of underlying energy forms, can be utilized as therapeutic patterning aids.

5. Viewing change as positive: The central focus of nursing is the phenomenon of unitary human beings in all their change processes. This includes aging and the dying process. For example, the words ''healthy'' and ''dying'' are not mutually exclusive. Nurses can assist the public and one another to accept death as a rhythmic phenomenon possessing its own inherent possibilites rather than as a negative condition to ward off as long as possible—that is, to experience a healthy death. Many American Indian tribes, for example, provided special places for their elders to go when they felt their times of death approaching. Many people desire to orchestrate their own deaths in terms of time, place, and those they want with them to mark their passage. This can be seen in the spread of the hospice as an alternative to hospitalization. Menstruation, pregnancy, menopause, and aging are other examples of change processes that are not pathological events, although often treated as such in other models.

A positive focus on change, manifested in correlates of patterning, all of which postulate development from lower frequency to higher frequency wave patterning of people from birth through old age, fosters a generalist approach to nursing practice on the graduate level. This is in contrast to clinical specialization, which tends to separate adult health from pediatrics, for example, and often sets psychiatric nursing apart from everything else.

6. *Expanding the assessment phase of the nursing process:* As an adjunct to physical assessment, nurses can do "nonphysical" assessments of the human energy field, using Therapeutic Touch to assess the rhythms and flow of energy. Because patterning is a dynamic process, assessments need to be performed on an ongoing basis in the context of field interactions.

7. *Accepting the integral connectedness of life:* This knowledge fosters social responsibility and concern for the health of the environment as inseparable from the health of humanity. This awareness is embedded within the Science of Unitary Human Beings; human and environment are inseparable and evolve together. For example, the healing milieu is as important as the healing modality. On a larger scale, there is a need for collective responsibility in the world where we are all interconnected.

The Science of Unitary Human Beings presents a new world view for nursing, one that requires a quantum leap from what we think we know to speculations about what might be. It suggests the total openness of experience, allowing us to reframe obstacles as opportunities. The dynamic, ever-changing dance of patterning with unitary human beings and their environments challenges us to find creative, innovative methods of practice.

The studies presented in the second half of this book offer insights into possibilities that exist for translating the framework into practice. Rawnsley investigates time perception, chronological age, and the dying process in hospitalized patients.[18] Ference has developed a tool to measure human field motion, the individual's perceptions in relation to feelings of "my motor is running" and "my field expansion," looking at human field motion in relation to time experience, creativity, and differentiation.[7] Malinski looks at hyperactive children from a perspective other than the traditional one.[15] McDonald explores the application of lightwaves (red and blue) to the hands of women with rheumatoid arthritis and assesses their perceptions of pain.[14] Cowling looks at indicators of pattern properties, examining the relationship of mystical experience, differentiation, and creativity in college students.[5] Alligood explores creativity, actualization, and empathy as indicators of the change process.[17] Gueldner examines imposed motion in the form of rocking, restedness, and the perception of human field motion with elderly nursing home residents.[8] Barrett defines power as "the capacity to participate knowingly in the nature of change characterizing the continuous repatterning of the human and environmental fields."[3] She has developed a set of scales to measure awareness, choices, freedom to act intentionally, and involvement in creating changes in relation to self, family, and occupation. Such studies can assist us in evolving our practice of nursing.

REFERENCES

1. Achterberg J, Lawlis F: Imagery and health intervention. Top Clin Nurs 1:55–60, 1982
2. ANA: Nursing, a Social Policy Statement. Kansas City, Mo, 1980
3. Barrett EAM: An Empirical Investigation of Martha E. Rogers' Principle of Helicy: The Relationship of Human Field Motion and Power, doctoral dissertation. New York University, 1983 (University Microfilms Publication No. 84–06, 278)
4. Cousins N: Anatomy of an Illness as Perceived by the Patient. New York, Bantam Books, 1981
5. Cowling R: The Relationship of Mystical Experience, Differentiation, and Creativity in College Students: An Empirical Investigation of the Principle of Helicy in Rogers' Science of Unitary Man, doctoral dissertation. New York University, 1982 (University Microfilms Publications No. 84–06, 283)
6. Fanslow C: Death: A natural facet of the life continuum. In Krieger D (ed): Foundations for Holistic Health Nursing Practices, The Renaissance Nurse. Philadelphia, Lippincott, 1981, pp 249–272
7. Ference H: The Relationship of Time Experience, Creativity Traits, Differentiation, and Human Field Motion, doctoral dissertation. New York University, 1979 (University Microfilms Publication No. 80–10, 281)
8. Gueldner SH: A Study of the Relationship Between Imposed Motion and Human Field Motion in Elderly Individuals Living in Nursing Homes, doctoral dissertation. University of Alabama in Birmingham, 1983 (University Microfilms Publication No. 83–20, 597)
9. Heidt P: Scientific research and therapeutic touch. In Borelli MD, Heidt P (eds): Therapeutic Touch. New York, Springer, 1981, pp 3–12
10. Krieger D: The Therapeutic Touch, How to Use Your Hands to Help or to Heal. Englewood Cliffs, NJ, Prentice-Hall, 1979
11. Krieger D: The creative nurse: A holistic perspective. In Krieger D (ed): Foundations for Holistic Health Nursing Practices, the Renaissance Nurse. Philadelphia, Lippincott, 1981, pp 137–148
12. LeShan L: You Can Fight for Your Life, Emotional Factors in the Treatment of Cancer. New York, M. Evans & Company, 1980
13. Macrae J: Therapeutic touch: A way of life. In Borelli MD, Heidt P (eds): Therapeutic Touch. New York, Springer, 1981, pp 49–58
14. McDonald SF: A Study of the Relationship Between Visible Lightwaves and the Experience of Pain, doctoral dissertation. Wayne State University, 1981 (University Microfilms Publication No. 81–17, 084)
15. Malinski VM: The Relationship Between Hyperactivity in Children and Perception of Short Wavelength Light: An Investigation into the Conceptual System Proposed by Dr. Martha E. Rogers, doctoral dissertation. New York University, 1980 (University Microfilms Publication No. 81–10, 669)
16. Quinn J: Therapeutic touch as energy exchange: Testing the theory. Adv Nurs Sci 6:42–49, 1984
17. Raile MM: The Relationship of Creativity, Actualization, and Empathy in Unitary Human Development: A Descriptive Study of Rogers' Principle of Helicy, doctoral dissertation. New York University, 1982 (University Microfilms Publication No. 83–13, 874)
18. Rawnsley MM: Relationships Between the Perception of the Speed of Time and the

Process of Dying: An Empirical Investigation of the Holistic Theory of Nursing Proposed by Martha Rogers, doctoral dissertation. Boston University School of Nursing, 1977 (University Microfilms No. 77–21, 692)

19. Rich A: Of Woman Born: Motherhood as Experience and Institution. New York, Norton, 1976
20. Rogers ME: Science of unitary human beings: A paradigm for nursing, 1983 (unpublished)
21. Rogers ME: Personal communication, 1984
22. Simonton OC, Matthews-Simonton S, Creighton JL: Getting Well Again. New York, Bantam, 1978
23. Starhawk: Dreaming in the Dark: Magic, Sex, and Politics. Boston, Beacon, 1982
24. Wurtman R: The effects of light on the human body. Sci Am 233:68–77, 1975

Part Two

Theory and Research

5

Foundations of a Nursing Science and Its Evolution: A Perspective

Helen M. Ference

Nursing has long been considered an art. The arts of caring for the sick, nurturing the healthy development of the young and the old, and promoting wellness have long been the themes of nursing. Although many schools of thought have emerged over the years, there is general agreement today, as in the past, that nurses care for the whole person.

Nursing's evolution as a science can be traced to the days of Nightingale, when patient data were collected and subjected to statistical tests for the purpose of determining probable outcomes. Nurses are avid observers and data collectors. Data collection techniques are inherent in the learning of systematic investigation of patients' health and the nursing process methodology. The specific data that are collected vary and are linked to phenomena of general interest to treatment givers from the respective eras of history.

Consider the nature of data collected by nurses in different eras and in different settings. For example, during the war years the assessment tools focused on physical injuries, physiological vital signs, reaction to treatment of wound care, and physiological healing. It could be observed in the postwar years, as nurses were increasingly employed by hospitals, that the emphasis on the data to be collected related to the reason for hospitalization. Data collection became easier once the medical diagnosis was determined. The medical diagnoses have aided us in developing specialty areas in nursing, such as surgical nursing, medical nursing, and cardiac nursing. These specialty areas have further assisted in narrowing the focus of our assessments. Today, observation is so specific that the forest cannot be seen because of the trees. In the process of observing the whole person, nursing has become expert in looking at the parts. It is time to reconsider the focus of nursing as the whole person.

This chapter will present a sketch of the emergence of that refocus and the shaping of that focus through research and theory development into the specific science of nursing, the Science of Unitary Human Beings.

SCOPE OF KNOWLEDGE

Observation has related to the scope of knowledge of nursing. The scope of knowledge can be traced to the nursing curricula. At one time, the fundamental courses in nursing generally were skills-related. This was especially true in the technical programs of nursing. When nursing moved into higher education, where baccalaureate degrees were considered entry-level to practice, there were prerequisite courses in related fields of anatomy, physiology, psychology, sociology, and chemistry. Nursing was considered an applied science, and the data collected related to nursing's knowledge of those related fields.

In the 1960s nursing experienced a revolution similar to those that were occurring in other segments of society. Nursing was coming into its own. In reaction to being a part of the academic world, nursing leaders raised questions such as: "What is nursing's domain?" "What theories are nursing theories?" and "Is there one theory of nursing?"

In the late 1960s and early 1970s, nursing programs were obliged to have curricula with nursing conceptual frameworks. Concept development became a natural part of thinking about nursing's domain. Concept development was a strategy used to shake up the traditional medical model, which was the current frame for nursing practice; rethink the phenomena that were of utmost importance in nursing practice; and restructure the phenomena within the curriculum and practice frameworks in order to focus on the insightful and new perspective. The entry-level programs in nursing that taught nursing within these new perspectives were called "integrated curricula." Their purpose was to teach all that was taught before, but teach it from a new perspective, a nursing model. Nursing had arrived. It publicly stated that it was different from medicine and that there were phenomena addressed only by students of the discipline of nursing.

This change was not an easy process. Nurse academicians who were secure in the traditions of the medical model reconceptualized phenomena of central concern to nursing. The orthopedic nurse focused on mobility–immobility, the critical care nurse focused on levels of dependence–independence, and the generalist attended to the whole person.

It was in this era of nursing's evolution that Rogers[39] synthesized the concepts of the Science of Unitary Human Beings and put forth a framework for the science and art of nursing that solely focused on the whole person in the continuous mutual process with the whole environmental field. A transformation in nursing was made. Nursing has never been the same since.

THE EARLY SCIENCE

The Rogerian framework, known originally as the Science of Unitary Man and more recently as the Science of Unitary Human Beings, was developed by Rogers during her years at New York University. The environment was well suited for this development. As head of the Division of Nursing, Rogers maintained the philosophy that nursing is both an art and a science and that nursing science focused on the whole person, a domain of study that was not addressed by any other discipline.

The setting was ideal. During the 1960s and the early 1970s there were few doctoral programs in nursing. New York University was one of the few universities with such a program, and therefore it served as a hub of scholarship and theory development for nursing's bright and inquisitive students. A master's program and undergraduate program also existed and allowed for a healthy mix of academicians, researchers, and clinicians.

As the faculty applied this early science for students, terminology was developed. In this developing era, there were references to "rhythms," which were often interpreted as body or physiological rhythms. There being no new data to collect yet, old indicators of body function rhythms, such as body temperature, were studied.

In Rogers' first publication of the framework,[39] she introduced the terms "field" and "field phenomena." The more evolved field was said to be expanded. There were four principles rather than the three proposed today. Reciprocy was changed to complimentarity and then integrality, and synchrony was dropped. The language of the science was emerging and with use was found either to bring specificity to the science or not to bring specificity. Words represent the phenomena of study, and the phenomena studied make up the class of facts for the science.

Determining the Class of Facts

The early studies were based upon some guiding assumptions and a philosophy that the nurse cares for the whole person. A retrospective analysis yields groupings of studies that investigated variables considered to be relevant to understanding the whole person. In the midsixties, there were studies of human development: Neal,[30] Porter,[35] and Earle.[11] Also, there were beginning studies of the "man"–environment interaction: Mathwig[27] and Felton.[14] In the 1970s, when Rogers was defining the principle of complementarity (now integrality), Bondy,[4] Cortes,[7] and Kissell[21] investigated variables of the environmental field in relation to the potentially relevant variables of the human field.

Studies of body image emerged in the late 1960s and continued through 1977: Warner,[47] Collett,[6] Olgas,[33] Fawcett,[13] Gordon,[18] Gioiella,[17] and Chodil,[5] in an effort to try to explain the perceptive reality of the human field and the environmental field. The image studies were crucial to the beginning interpretations of reality in a four-dimensional perspective, in contrast to the manifestations of the field, which are considered reality in a three-dimensional perspective.

At the time of most of these studies the term "boundaries" was being used. There was an effort to explain the border or boundaries between the human and environmental fields. In the late 1970s, Rogers discontinued the use of the word "boundaries," explaining that it did not clarify what it was intended to clarify. According to the Science of Unitary Human Beings, the human and environmental energy fields are in continuous mutual process—complementarity, as defined by Rogers.[40, 41] The human field boundary was becoming a focus of investigation rather than the continuous mutual process of the fields. Although this distinction may seem slight, it serves as an example of how language can bring meaning to phenomena.

In the early to mid-1970s, there were several nursing studies conducted about the variable of time. Rather than assume the relative space–time factor of the Rogerian framework, many scientists set out to test Rogers' postulation that time moves quickly with high frequency energy, in an effort to explain the phenomenon's relationship to the human field. These were early studies, so it must be remembered that often there was no specific reference to the person as an energy field. Often there is little reference to the framework, aside from a quote of an assumption or guiding principle. Time perception was described according to its relationship with gait tempo by Newman,[32] temporal orientation and extension by Fitzpatrick,[16] and rate of speech and listening by Boguslawski.[3] Time estimation was studied with light wave frequency by Nelson,[31] and judgment of time duration was investigated with field independence and posture by Phillips.[34] These studies helped future researchers to define the meaning of time in a space–time context.

The studies of locus of control, field independence, and differentiation contributed to a better understanding of the differences between psychological differentiation and the phenomenon of concern in the Rogerian framework postulated to be human field differentiation. Early 1970s studies, Holley,[20] Barnard,[1] Miller,[29] Dirschel,[10] Swanson,[45] and Falco,[12] often specified an assumption of the Science of Unitary Human Beings but relied on the theories of other disciplines, particularly psychology, to frame the hypotheses.

Science evolves. The contributions of many scientists bring new insights through the testing and retesting of phenomena that are central to the concern of the particular science. In this case the phenomenon of concern is the unitary human.

Kuhn[22] has identified three normal foci or "classes of problems" that are inherent in a scientific paradigm. Determining the significant class of facts is the first focus. The evolution that has thus far been described for the Science of Unitary Human Beings shows that struggle. The second is "matching of facts with theory," and the third is the "articulation of the theory." The second focus took hold in 1977 and continues today.

Matching Facts with Theory

In 1977, Rawnsley, of Boston University, framed her research solely within the Rogerian framework.[37] This study marked a turning point for research in the Science of Unitary Human Beings. For the first time, hypotheses were derived from the Rogerian conceptual framework. Until this time assumptions of the framework were stated in the research reports, but many of the theoretical frameworks were logically constructed of theories from many sciences other than nursing. In a strict interpretation, it may be said that there was no research in the framework prior to 1977. However, some of the variables that were under investigation prior to that time were relevant for study in the framework. The search for facts became easier when the research was framed solely by the complete framework.

Not being from New York University, Rawnsley had an advantage and a disadvantage. The disadvantage was her absence from the frequent updating sessions by Rogers regarding changes in the terminology. This disadvantage actually served as a blessing in disguise, because it forced Rawnsley to rely mainly on Rogers' original publication of the framework.[39] By 1977 it was found that certain aspects of the framework did not serve to clarify it, such as the principle of synchronicity. Reading Rawnsley's report of a study framed in the 1970 version of the Science of "Man" confirmed the need for changes, which by 1977 were in process at New York University, but not yet published. Thus Rawnsley's report was an advantage to the many doctoral students engaged in frequent, scholarly discussions about testing theories derived specifically from the Rogerian framework.

It was with this background that the present author set out to specify Rogers' correlates of development, operationally defining them so that they were mutually exclusive, in order to subject them to empirical test. The first instrument, Ference's Human Field Motion Test, was developed in 1978, piloted, and then used with other revalidated instruments to test the construct validity of the correlates of synergistic human development.[15]

Many studies followed. Human field motion has been investigated with the variables of sensation seeking (Lindley),[23] imposed motion of the elderly (Gueldner),[19] meditation (MacCrae),[25] power (Barrett),[2] and red and blue light and blindness (Ludomirski-Kalmanson).[24] Other studies are in process by faculty at Case Western Reserve University[9] and the University of Tennessee in Memphis.[46]

The subsequent studies at New York University that were testing theories derived from the Rogerian framework clearly specified that as the intention: Cowling,[8] Raile,[36] Reeder,[38] Malinski,[26] Miller,[28] Sarter,[42] and Barrett.[2] In fact, some specify that a principle of the framework is being tested, such as the principle of helicy: Barrett[2] and Raile.[36]

In 1983, a second instrument was developed and reported as a measure of the whole person. Barrett's Human Field Power Test[2] is a measure of the capacity to participate knowingly in change. Thus far, human field power correlates with human field motion as two distinguishing features of unitary humans. Barrett's Power Test is being used by researchers at the University of Tennessee at Memphis[43] and at Case Western University.[44]

The Science of Unitary Human Beings has the three classes of problems that Kuhn describes in the structure of science. It is no longer appropriate to mix theoretical frameworks or to borrow theories from other sciences while investigating the theories of the Science of Unitary Human Beings. At the time of this writing it can be said that "work under the paradigm can be conducted in no other way, and to desert the paradigm is to cease practicing the science it defines."[22]

ROGERIAN PHILOSOPHY OR ROGERIAN SCIENCE

In the developing years of the Rogerian framework there were other theoretical frameworks emerging in nursing. There was a common reaction to treat these frameworks as philosophies, or belief systems. This nonscientific view limits the potential development and use of the Rogerian framework.

The Rogerian framework is a science. It is the science of nursing, referred to as the Science of Unitary Human Beings. Webster's *Third New International Dictionary* defines a science as "a department of systematized knowledge as an object of study or knowledge attained through study or practice."[48] This framework differs from others in its conceptual base and its demand of studying a specific body of knowledge. There is a basic knowledge that must be acquired before full integration of learning can occur. The understanding of new physics and four-dimensionality are paramount.

Much of the research conducted specifically in the Science of Unitary Human Beings is basic research. "Basic research" generally refers to the discovery and explanation of new phenomena. This type of research contrasts with clinical research, where problems are identified and explanations are sought for purposes of remedy.

Basic research often has no associated values. Often we do not know whether we like or do not like a finding. Consequently, the finding is given a "So what?" or "Who cares?" by the quick-fix professional. Serious students of the discipline must devote their time to observing such phenomena, for it is through this intense and inquisitive, systematic investigation that we begin to see that which has gone unnoticed before. When a new phenomenon is seen clearly, there can be beginning observations and associations defined with old phenomena that are already identified as problems or, in some instances, as health-related assets.

A Specific Language

A science has a language of specificity. The evolution of a science is a slow process. It demands the learning of a new language. From the architects of the science it demands drafting, testing, and rewriting the language in order that the words mean what they are intended to mean.

Rogers is, of course, the primary source for maintaining an update of terminology as it changes. However, it is possible to assure a continuity by using the definitions that have been used by researchers in their respective studies. At this point in the development of the science, new operational definitions should not be used unless the researcher logically assesses the previous definitions and assertively offers an alternative. This logical redefinition should be conducted with reference to the assumptions and principles of the Rogerian framework. If there is a failure to build theoretical and operational definitions in this way, it will be most difficult to justify the interconnection of the framework and support construct development.

Over the years there have been terminology changes. Many have been mentioned in this chapter, such as "rhythms," "boundary," "field expansion," "reciprocity," and "synchronicity." Many of the changes were made when terms did not bring clarification to understanding the human field in a four-dimensional perspective. A glossary is provided in this book. Also, definitions are available in the original reports of the studies reported herein.

SUMMARY

The value of reflection is meaning. Reflection on the development of the Science of Unitary Human Beings provides the opportunity to make sense out of a series of actions, put the events in place for posterity, and move on to a greater understanding and participation in the pattern of science. From a four-dimensional perspective, this reflection is in fact an insightful image of reality that emerges with synthesis, a pattern transformation.

The object of this chapter has not been to speak the language of four-dimensionality. Rather, it has been an attempt to bring meaning to the nature of the Science of Unitary Human Beings. The experience of learning this new language is like sitting on the border of a new country. First, we are inquisitive. Second, we learn a few words. Third, we realize that some of our old concepts are absent in this new language and that some new concepts are present. Fourth, we develop an understanding of thinking, a new perspective that relates to our fluency in the language. And, fifth, a synthesis has been reached and the new language is integrated into our daily lives. We have become bilingual. We now are fluent in our old and new languages.

And so, when we live in a bilingual world, as is often necessary for the scientists of the Rogerian framework, we must be ever mindful of speaking the language that relates to the synthesis of four-dimensionality, openness, whole energy fields, and related pattern manifestations. The object of our research must clearly be derived from the framework. Scientific methods are merely tools for bringing explanation and understanding to the phenomena of investigation.

The technology of our three-dimensional world and the mathematical models can serve to help us see the phenomenon of the whole person. There are technology and mathematical models that are compatible with the Rogerian framework. However, it is imperative that we not lose sight of the indices of wholeness by placing our primary attention on methodologies. The methodologies are a means to an end. The end is the outcome of our science and our research. It is the description and explanation of the whole person. In order to achieve that end, we must continue to explicate the theories in the framework. We must also use the tools that were designed as measures of the four-dimensional field.

We must continually link our research to theory and articulate the theories. It is this broader conceptual linkage that provides our broad perspective of the whole person and forms our nursing science. It is through our research derived from this framework that we will make fundamental contributions to the general science of human beings. In this way, nursing will serve humanity through its knowledge. The knowledge will not only be applicable in our small world of nursing practice. It will be basic to the fundamental understanding of humankind.

REFERENCES

1. Barnard R: Field Independence–Dependence and Selected Motor Abilities, doctoral dissertation. New York University, 1973 (University Microfilms)
2. Barrett EAM: An Empirical Investigation of Rogers' Principle of Helicy: The Relationship of Human Field Complexity, Human Field Motion and Power, doctoral dissertation. New York University, 1983 (University Microfilms)
3. Boguslawski M: An Investigation of the Relationship Between Speech Rate, Preferred Listening Rate of Speech and Perception of Time, doctoral dissertation, New York University, 1975 (University Microfilms)
4. Bondy K: An Investigation Through Semantic Encoding of the Differences in Selected Environmental Events by Varying Shape and Motion, doctoral dissertation. New York University, 1975 (University Microfilms)
5. Chodil J: An Investigation of the Relation Between Perceived Body Space, Actual Body Space, Body Image Boundary, and Self Esteem (Research Study). Funded in part by Sigma Theta Tau Research Grant, 1977–1978
6. Collett B: A Study of the Relationship Between Variation in Body Temperature, Perceived Duration and Perceived Personal Space, doctoral dissertation. New York University, 1972 (University Microfilms)
7. Cortes T: An Investigation of the Relationship Between Lightwaves and Cardiac Rate, doctoral dissertation. New York University, 1975 (University Microfilms)
8. Cowling WR: The Relationship of Mystical Experience, Differentiation, and Creativity in College Students: An Empirical Investigation of the Principle of Helicy in Rogers' Science of Unitary Man, doctoral dissertation. New York University, 1982 (University Microfilms)
9. Cowling WR, Vines S: The Relationship of Age to Rogers' Correlates of Development. Study in process at Case Western Reserve University, Frances Payne Bolton School of Nursing, 1985
10. Dirschel K: The Relationship of Field Dependence–Independence and Cultural Conformity to Attitudes Toward the Aged in Selected Nursing Students, doctoral dissertation. New York University, 1974 (University Microfilms)
11. Earle A: The Effect of Supplementary Postnatal Kinesthetic Stimulation on the Developmental Behavior of the Normal Female Newborn, doctoral dissertation. New York University, 1969 (University Microfilms)
12. Falco S: The Relationship Between Field Dependence, Visual Output, and Gross Motor Activity in Individuals Confined to Bed, doctoral dissertation. New York University, 1975 (University Microfilms)
13. Fawcett J: The Relationship Between Spouses' Strength of Identification and their Patterns of Change in Perceived Body Space and Articulation of Body Concept During and After Pregnancy, doctoral dissertation. New York University, 1976 (University Microfilms)
14. Felton G: A Study of the Relationship Between an Abrupt One Hour Shift in the Social Routine and the Extent of Duration of Blood Pressure and Temperature Changes in Young Women, doctoral dissertation. New York University, 1968 (University Microfilms)

15. Ference HM: The Relationship of Time Experience, Creativity Traits, Differentiation, and Human Field Motion: An Empirical Investigation of Rogers' Correlates of Synergistic Human Development, doctoral dissertation. New York University, 1979 (University Microfilms)

16. Fitzpatrick JJ: An Investigation of the Relationship Between Temporal Orientation, Temporal Extension and Time Perception, doctoral dissertation. New York University, 1975 (University Microfilms)

17. Gioiella E: The Relationships Between Slowness of Response, State Anxiety, Social Isolation and Self Esteem and Preferred Personal Space in the Elderly, doctoral dissertation. New York University, 1977 (University Microfilms)

18. Gordon S: Relationships Among Anxiety, Expressed Satisfaction with Body Image and Maladaptive Physiological Responses in Pregnancy, doctoral dissertation. New York University, 1976 (University Microfilms)

19. Gueldner S: A Study of the Relationship Between Imposed Motion and Human Field Motion in Elderly Individuals Living in Nursing Homes, doctoral dissertation. University of Alabama in Birmingham, 1983 (University Microfilms)

20. Holley M: Field Independence–Dependence, Sophistication-of-Body-Concept in Social Distance Selection, doctoral dissertation. New York University, 1972 (University Microfilms)

21. Kissell P: The Relationship of Self Esteem, Programmed Music, and Time of Day to Preferred Conversational Distance among Female College Students, doctoral dissertation. New York University, 1974 (University Microfilms)

22. Kuhn T: The Structure of Scientific Revolutions, 2nd ed. Chicago, University of Chicago Press, 1970

23. Lindley PA: An Empirical Study of the Relationship of Sensation Seeking to the Human Energy Field Motion Within Rogers' Science of Unitary Man, master's thesis. University of Rochester, 1981

24. Ludormirski-Kalmanson B: Relationship Between the Environmental Energy Wave Frequency Pattern Manifest in Red Light and Blue Light and Human Field Motion in Adult Individuals with Visual Sensory Perception and Those With Total Blindness, doctoral dissertation. New York University, 1984 (University Microfilms)

25. Macrae J: A Comparison Between Meditating Subjects and Non-Meditating Subjects on Time Experience and Human Field Motion, doctoral dissertation. New York University, 1982 (University Microfilms)

26. Malinski V: The Relationship Between Hyperactivity in Children and Perception of Short Wavelength Light: An Investigation into the Conceptual System Proposed by Martha E. Rogers, doctoral dissertation. New York University, 1980 (University Microfilms)

27. Mathwig G: Living Open Systems, Reciprocal Adaptations and the Life Process, doctoral dissertation. New York University, 1967 (University Microfilms)

28. Miller F: The Relationship of Sleep, Wakefulness, and Beyond Waking Experience: A Descriptive Study of M. Rogers' Concept of Sleep-Wake Rhythm, doctoral dissertation. New York University, 1984 (University Microfilms)

29. Miller S: An Investigation of the Relationship Between Mothers' General Fearfulness, Their Daughters' Locus of Control, and General Fearfulness in the Daughter, doctoral dissertation. New York University, 1974 (University Microfilms)

30. Neal M: The Relationship Between a Regimen of Vestibular Stimulation and Developmental Behavior of the Small Premature Infant, doctoral dissertation. New York University, 1967 (University Microfilms)

31. Nelson M: An Investigation of the Relationship of Visible Light Wave Frequencies and

Man's Time Estimation, doctoral dissertation. New York University, 1975 (University Microfilms)

32. Newman M: An Investigation of the Relationship Between Gait Tempo and Time Perception, doctoral dissertation. New York University, 1971 (University Microfilms)

33. Olgas M: The Relationship Between Parents' Health Status and Body Image of Their Children, doctoral dissertation. New York University, 1973 (University Microfilms)

34. Phillips J: An Investigation of the Relationship Between Field Dependence-Independence, Posture, and Judgement of Time Duration, doctoral dissertation. New York University, 1976 (University Microfilms)

35. Porter L: Physical-Physiological Activity and Infants' Growth and Development, doctoral dissertation. New York University, 1967 (University Microfilms)

36. Raile M: The Relationship of Creativity, Actualization, and Empathy in Unitary Human Development: A Descriptive Study of Rogers' Principle of Helicy, doctoral dissertation. New York University, 1982 (University Microfilms)

37. Rawnsley M: Relationships Between the Perception of the Speed of Time and the Process of Dying: An Empirical Investigation of the Holistic Theory of Nursing Proposed by Martha Rogers, doctoral dissertation. Boston University, 1977 (University Microfilms)

38. Reeder F: Nursing Research, Holism, and Philosophies of Science: Points of Congruence Between Edmund Husserl and Martha E. Rogers, doctoral dissertation. New York University, 1984 (University Microfilms)

39. Rogers M: An Introduction to the Theoretical Basis of Nursing. Philadelphia, F. A. Davis, 1970

40. Rogers M, Ference H: Modification of the definition of the principle of complementarity. Class handout, Deriving Testable Hypotheses from the Science of Unitary Man, New York University Division of Nursing, October 1979

41. Rogers M: Nursing science: A science of unitary human beings, November 22, 1982 (unpublished paper of terminology)

42. Sarter B: The Stream of Becoming: A Metaphysical Analysis of Rogers' Model of Unitary Man, doctoral dissertation. New York University, 1984 (University Microfilms)

43. Scandrett S: The indigenous healing process, University of Tennessee Center for the Health Sciences, College of Nursing, 1985 (in progress)

44. Segall M: Health conception, locus of control, and power as indicators of life style change. Case Western Reserve University, Frances Payne Bolton School of Nursing, 1985 (in progress)

45. Swanson A: An Investigation of the Relationship Between a Child's General Fearfulness and the Child's Mother's Anxiety, Self Differentiation, and Accuracy of Perception of Her Child's General Fearfulness, doctoral dissertation. New York University, 1975 (University Microfilms)

46. Thomas S: The experience of intentionality and human field motion: A test of the principle of integrality according to the Rogerian framework. University of Tennessee Center for the Health Sciences, College of Nursing, 1985 (in progress)

47. Warner B: The Relationship Between Reported Self and Body Image Satisfaction and Attitudes Toward Aging of Senior Nursing Students Enrolled in Hospital Schools of Nursing, doctoral dissertation. New York University, 1969 (University Microfilms)

48. Webster's Third New, International Dictionary, unabridged. Springfield, Mass, Merriam, 1976

6

Basic Theoretical Research in the Conceptual System of Unitary Human Beings

Francelyn Reeder

Theory development derived from the Rogerian conceptual system of unitary human beings warrants extensive scholarship on metascientific evaluation criteria for assessing theories. Lauden, a contemporary philosopher of science, observes that "the views of the scientific community about how to test theories and about what counts as evidence have changed dramatically through history."[7] This chapter, based on a philosophical study,[11] focuses on the congruence between evaluative criteria for assessing knowledge and the Rogerian conceptual system. Congruence between basic assumptions undergirding these two intellectual tools is crucial to logical and relevant theory development for nursing as a field of inquiry. The net gain from an application of such a philosophical test of congruence (1) manifests substantial clarification and understanding of the central phenomena of interest to nursing, (2) identifies the nature of knowledge ascribed by the phenomena of unitary human beings, and (3) illuminates the role of the scientist required in the access and evaluation of these phenomena.

Specifically, the following types of analyses were utilized to accomplish the goals of this basic theoretical research in the Rogerian conceptual system:

1. Explication and concept–contextual analyses of basic assumptions of the Rogerian conceptual system that point to the nature and acquisition of knowledge of unitary human beings (the phenomenon of interest)
2. Explication and concept–contextual analyses of basic assumptions of phenomenology (Husserlian) that indicate the scope of phenomena accessible to investigation through multiple modes of human awareness
3. Selection of one postulate among the basic assumptions of Rogerian science and one from the principal assumptions of phenomenology for exploration of congruence between the two

In the following section these major postulates are presented first from the author's perspective and then are explored for points of congruency.

FOUR-DIMENSIONALITY IN THE ROGERIAN CONCEPTUAL SYSTEM

The focus of the Rogerian conceptual system is *unitary human beings* which means that human beings are integral with the environment (all that is other than itself).[23] Rogers specifies four building blocks in the conceptual system, which are: (1) energy fields, (2) open systems, (3) pattern, and (4) four-dimensionality.

After reading and reflecting on Rogers' writings available in print between 1961 to 1983, the author found that the persistent building block commanding attention for reasons of its appeal as a potential humanizing characteristic was that of four-dimensionality. Four-dimensionality, more than any of the other three building blocks, is of interest to the discussion of holism because it indicates the nature and process of knowledge required of this system.[11, 15, 18, 20, 21] The evidence required is a knowledge realm distinct from three-dimensional sense-perceptible evidence required in natural science.[4]

This building block also is more fully described with linkages to the rest of the conceptual system than the others and therefore considered more accessible to explicate. This, however, does not mean it is necessarily easier to understand. Of equal importance, four-dimensionality remains the building block about which most questions are asked by scholars in nursing.[22, 24]

Explication of Four-Dimensionality in the Writings of Rogers

"Four-dimensionality" first appeared as a specific term in 1979.[18] However, rudiments can be identified in earlier writings in general discussions of the characteristics of "living systems"[17] and the "life process in man"[15].

Discussion of four-dimensionality began in 1970 with Rogers'[17] major text as it reads:

> Envision the human field embedded in the curvature of space-time. The life process is the expression of the rhythmical evolution of the field along a spiralling longitudinal axis, bound in the four-dimensional space-time matrix and ever shaped and being shaped by the environment. The human field occupies space, extending in all directions. The field projects into the future as well as into the past. The creativity of life emerges out of the man-environment interaction along life's continuum. The human field is continually adding new dimensions of growing complexity, evidenced in life's negentropic qualities (p. 91).[17]

In 1970[17] Rogers cited Einstein's Theory of Relativity as a point of intrigue specifically as it expressed a new concept of four-dimensionality derived from a synthesis of three-dimensional space with time. Rogers[23] has said on numerous occasions that she does not build on Einstein's concept of four-dimensionality per se but rather uses it as a stimulus for further questions about human and environment relationships.

For example, Einstein[5] conceived of the Theory of Relativity after realizing the integral role the scientist's perception plays in the phenomena studied. It can be said that a paradoxical nature of the scientist is expressed in Einstein's conceptualizing of the integral role of the knower and the known while also recognizing that the knower is capable of realizing this integral relationship as such.

Likewise, Rogers expresses her conception of unitary human beings integral with the environment yet somehow striving beyond to understand and see another view: "Man moves to transcend himself. A scenario comes into view."[21]

Rogers further synthesized the notion of four-dimensionality and conceived of it as one of the four building blocks of her conceptual system in 1979.[18] For example, Rogers depicted four-dimensionality for the first time with Figure 6–1.

As Rogers presents four-dimensionality, she suggests that, for adequate schematization of this concept, "substantial abstract thinking" is required.[18] Rogers also reminds the reader that four-dimensionality postulates a world "of neither space nor time," as these concepts are used by Newtonian science.[18] Further, Rogers invites readers to use their imagination and refers them to an analogy in Abbott's *Flatland*.[1] Both were to be used as aids to the understanding and conceptualizing of four-dimensionality. Rogers suggests that, while looking at Figure 6–1, one "imagine unitary man as a four-dimensional energy field embedded in a four-dimensional environmental field."[18]

In this imaginary view,

the four-dimensional human field is characterized by continuously fluctuating imaginary boundaries. The present as a point in time is not relevant to a 4-D model. Rather the four-dimensional human field is the "relative present" for any individual. . . . Four-dimensional reality is perceived as a synthesis of non-linear coordinates from which innovative change continuously and evolutionally emerges (p. 4).[18]

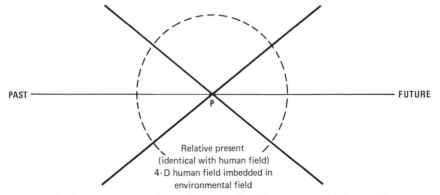

Figure 6–1. Rogers' postulate of four-dimensionality. *(From Rogers, 1979, p. 3.[18])*

After presenting all four building blocks, Rogers states they "are integral to the imaginative synthesis out of which a conceptual system emerges."[18] In other words, imaginative synthesis is integral to the building blocks (constructs) of (1) open systems, (2) energy fields, (3) pattern, and (4) four-dimensionality. These four, viewed together in a synthetic process, are said to form the basis from which a conceptual system emerges.[18] Thus, the development of the conceptual system of unitary human beings presented by Rogers implies, first, a beginning point of synthesized reality of facts and ideas and, secondly, imaginative synthesis from this synthesizing reality, which gives rise to a new product: the conceptual system of unitary human beings.

The central focus while developing a conceptual system representative of unitary human beings is also from the perspective of unitary human beings. The construct of unitary human being itself is a type, specifically, of a holistic construct, which Rogers postulates is "a synergistic phenomenon whose behaviors cannot be predicted by knowledge of the parts."[18]

Rogers states this postulate but does not explicitly state how she came to this conceptualization of unitary human beings. However, it can be inferred from further descriptors of four-dimensionality integral to the conceptual system that the same kind of imaginative synthesis advocated in the development of the conceptual system is also the process actually used by Rogers in the development of the original constructs and building blocks of the system. With such a view, it is suggested that the type of holism postulated by Rogers is synthesized from her self-given processes.

Additional descriptors of four-dimensionality have been given elsewhere by Rogers. These clarify the meaning ascribed by her in contradistinction to the use of four-dimensionality in other disciplines. For example, Rogers states:

> The four-dimensionality of which I speak is not a spatial dimension nor is it to be confused with the 4th dimensions being proposed by other disciplines such as mathematics and psychology. A four-dimensional world is clearly different from a three-dimensional world (p. 3).[18]

In a further elaboration of four-dimensionality, in which "human field" and "relative present" are discussed, Rogers states they are "identical" and as central concepts within four-dimensionality become helpful in "explaining paranormal events."[18] Specifically, Rogers explains:

> Clairvoyance . . . is rational in a four-dimensional human field in continuous mutual, simultaneous interaction with a four-dimensional environmental field. So too are such events as psychometry, therapeutic touch, telepathy and a wide range of other phenomena. Within this conceptual system such behaviors become "normal" rather than "paranormal (p. 6)."[18]

She points out that "what is a 'relative present' for one person is different from that of someone else."[18]

These are extreme examples; nonetheless, they make the point that phenomena other than three-dimensional, sensory experiences actually occur for humans and therefore indicate a capacity of human awareness not accounted for in a three-dimensional world view. This capacity is one that needs to be accounted for in a science of unitary human beings.[17]

Human experiences of an ordinary nature that are also different from three-dimensional reality are discussed by Rogers as needing investigation from a different perspective. She states,

Man's feelings and thoughts are not limited to the waking state. . . . Dreams provide a further means whereby integration and patterning of life occur (p. 72).[17]

The concept of time is another point of distinction in the building block of four-dimensionality. Rogers indicates two kinds of time that humans experience; "time passing is clearly different from time estimation."[17] Further, the nature of the "relative present" is expressed by Rogers as "the infinite now" in the following:

Rhythmicities of extraordinary complexity weave pulsating patterns through threads of yesteryear and the "infinite now" expands (p. 1).[20]

In 1981, more refinement is evident in expressions about four-dimensionality by Rogers:

Four-dimensionality is a non-linear domain without spatial or temporal attributes. The real world is postulated to be four-dimensional. The present as a point in time has no place in this paradigm. Rather the four-dimensional human field is the "relative present" or "infinite now" for any individual (p. 2).[20]

She further refines the concept of four-dimensionality by stating:

Indeed, the human field is synonymous with relative present. Each human field is unique and so too is the infinite now coordinate with any given human field. This is not a contradiction of multidimensionality. Rather it specifies that the real world is four-dimensional and other dimensions are abstractions (p. 222).[24]

"Energy field" is a construct used in the definition of four-dimensionality as a "unifying concept."[18] Clarification of this term is therefore necessary to understand other aspects of four-dimensionality. Energy field is a unifying concept and is

postulated to constitute the fundamental unit of both the living and the non-living. Field is a unifying concept. Energy signifies the dynamic nature of the field. Energy fields are unbounded. Two energy fields are identified: the human field and the environmental field. Specifically man and environment are energy fields.

They do not have energy fields. The unitary human field is not a biological field, or a physical field, or a social field, or a psychological field. Unitary man has his own integrity (p. 2).[18]

The general context of four-dimensionality is always the conceptual system of unitary human beings as a whole. Rogers frequently states the development of such a system "cannot be merely by a process of arrangements";[15] accordingly, she suggests that "it seeks to push back the frontiers of knowledge and those who seek to push back frontiers must have come close to those frontiers themselves."[15]

Although poetic (perhaps necessarily poetic), these lines point to a broad range of human experience to gain access to new knowledge. Elsewhere, Rogers[11, 15, 19] has frequently indicated ways to push back the frontiers of knowledge, one of them being through "imaginative synthesis." In this context, Rogers further comments that "this is not to suggest that one must know all the multiplicity of facts that have accumulated through the ages."[15] Rather, and she quotes Jacques Barzun for emphasis,

[t]he difficulty today is not that science has uncovered more facts than one mind can retain but that science has ceased to be, even to scientists, a set of principles and an object of contemplation (p. 42).[15]

Such an emphasis indicates another way to push back the frontiers of knowledge and includes reflection upon the conceptual system of unitary human beings, a standing back to gain perspective concomitantly with an integral view of human and environmental fields in mutual process. As the discussion began on four-dimensionality, so too does it come to a close with reference to the paradoxical nature of knowing required in the conceptual system of unitary human beings. That is, the knower and the known are integral and multidimensional, manifesting this integrality and diversity simultaneously.

Upon closer examination of four-dimensionality in the context of the whole system of unitary human beings from a phenomenological perspective, a congruence becomes apparent between two respective basic postulates: specifically, four-dimensionality in the Rogerian conceptual system and the principle of intentionality in Husserlian phenomenology.

The congruence is first evident in the problems and issues that led to Rogers' development of the concept of holism present in her conceptual system of unitary human beings. For example, it can be said that a motive force behind four-dimensionality as a construct derives from a felt need to sidestep the atomistic view of humans in the environment, a view expressed by Rogers as "knowledge of the whole cannot be predicted from knowledge of the parts."[22] It is a step toward replacing the prevailing philosophy of science preference for analyzing the parts and then summing them up to make a whole in an additive way.

However, from a reflective stance, the same question can be asked of Rogers as Husserl asked of the writings of James, Hume, and Descartes. That is, how do we deal with the problem of the possibility of knowledge of the whole if not through the parts? It is not logical to start with an assumption of wholeness. Rather, the assumption needs to be investigated for its very possibility. How can knowledge of the whole otherwise come about?

This problem is akin to the problem of identity recognized by numerous philosophers. The problem of identity concerns the possibility of identity of the same object through a multiplicity of acts or manifestations, and is discussed in this study under the heading "Principle of Intentionality." For a detailed account see the dissertation by Reeder.[11]

EXPLICATION OF THE PRINCIPLE OF INTENTIONALITY (UNITY OF INNER-TIME-CONSCIOUSNESS OF THE WORLD)

Access to Integral Evidence Through a Holistic Epistemology

Transcendental phenomenology (Husserlian) is an integrated way of philosophizing that derives and is derived from a rigorous investigation of the essential structure of consciousness of the world (C-W). One, it is the foundation of the "life-world" *(Lebenswelt)*. Two, the problem of identity of the same object (transcendental consciousness here) throughout a multiplicity of modes of awareness is achieved in Husserl's description of inner-time-consciousness as nontemporal, nonspatial, and noncausal. Three, the nature of syntheses as explicated is different from Kant's productive imagination of objects. Four, the multiple modes of awareness possible for the intending of any object are described more fully than any philosophy of science achieved before Husserl.

Figure 6–2 (principle of intentionality) provides a guide to the description of inner-time-consciousness. It is designed to indicate the dynamic, diverse, tentative nature of knowledge in which identity (unity) obtains throughout a multiplicity of modes of awareness. It depicts consciousness of the world as always integral, and as constituting and being constituted as the same throughout a multiplicity of modes of awareness of objects. The nonlinear nature of inner-time-consciousness is founded in the "Now" position of intentions directed to possible and actual objects through multiple modes of awareness. Furthermore, C-W in the "Now" is likewise retending* objects actually intended in the "Now" and also protending possible objects.

Several characteristics describe inner-time-consciousness of the world. First, the constituting C-W is not an "egoic" consciousness of a particular individual located in space and time, but rather universal, general consciousness. That is,

---

* The term "retending" used by Husserl describes the founding conditions for the possibility of egoic memory. It is one type of intending constituting the unity of inner-time-consciousness along with protending and intending from the "Now" position. "Protending" describes the founding conditions for the possibility of egoic expectation and anticipation.[8]

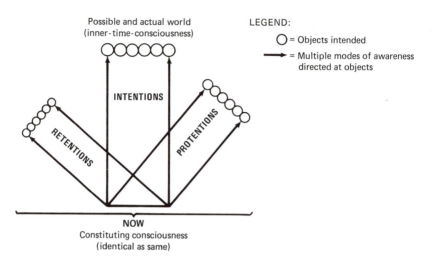

Figure 6–2. Principle of intentionality in phenomenology (consciousness of the world always integral). *(Resources: Gurwitsch,[6] Wiggins,[28] Design: Reeder.[11])*

such a constituting C-W describes the essential structures and functions of consciousness for its possibility as such, no matter what form it takes.

Husserl described such a universal constituting C-W grasped through intellectual intuition after performing the requirements for a phenomenological perspective; that is, as a result of performing the "transcendental epoche" and the "eidetic (essential) epoche" commonly referred to as "bracketing" the world. It involves an "unbuilding" process from the everyday way of experiencing the world as sense-perceptible and actual to a way of experiencing the world as possible and intelligible through reflection, intellectual intuition, and imagination.*

In such a domain C-W is nonspatial, nontemporal, and noncausal, yet intelligible. The categories of space, time, and causality, which Kant claimed were necessary conditions for the possibility of knowledge, on the contrary were not grasped or found by Husserl in the transcendental perspective of the C-W. Therefore, not given in firsthand (apodictive evidence), Husserl cannot affirm these categories as necessary to all experiences of the world.

In contrast, verification of the conceivable and imaginable inner-time-consciousness was not contradicted by further phenomenological evidence and, thus, accordingly was affirmed by Husserl.[8] Yet, this knowledge is held as tentative, always capable of being contradicted by further evidence. Knowledge of C-W is open and evolving, dynamic, and diverse. Through this tentative, changing diversity of C-W the identity of transcendental consciousness is given again and again into infinity.

---

* Transcendental epoche and eidetic epoche are essential to Husserlian phenomenological investigation and are described in detail in the following section entitled "Modes of Gaining Access to Integral Evidence in Transcendental Phenomenology."

Modes of Gaining Access to Integral Evidence in Transcendental Phenomenology

The following modes of gaining access to integral evidence C-W are described in the epistemology of Husserl. The first two modes make possible the others: (1) constitution (syntheses) of various types; (2) multiple modes of awareness of actual and possible objects; (3) reflection, in which objects are constituted as "my world;" (4) the transcendental epoche and eidetic epoche to temporarily set aside preconceived or scientific explanations of the world; (5) intellectual as well as sensible intuition; (6) imagination of nonsensible as well as sensible possibilities; (7) conceptualization of possible and actual realities; (8) imaginative variation of actual or possible objects, correlative with multiple modes of awareness; (9) synthesis of identification by which the essential structures of objects as intended are grasped (the identity throughout the multiplicity becomes apparent); (10) recognition of essential relations between identities. These essential relations obtain in the investigation of thematized objects (objects focused on).

Furthermore, the phenomenological method described by Husserl derives and is derived from the syntheses inherent in inner-time-consciousness, which signify our access to all objectivity of the world as known. Constitution is synonymous with synthesis in the principle of intentionality (Husserl).[8] Conversely, synthesis is not a process of analysis of parts followed by an effort to unify them by reason, but in its rudimentary forms it varies from being passive (automatic) to being active (egoless activity) correlative with the domains accessed through the multiple modes of awareness. Three types of syntheses are described in the dynamic nature of inner-time-consciousness.

Types of Synthesis

Husserl describes a certain order among the mutliple modes of awareness that obtain on the bases of prior dynamic processes. Husserl[8] noted one clue to this order in William James' reference to "bifocal awareness" in which a "focus" and a "fringe" are noticed in experience. The fringe is generally taken for granted but is the background of anything focused on or given attention.

The continuity of nature is taken for granted in everyday experience and by natural science.[6] In the quest for meaning Husserl tries to explicate the possible conditions for the possibility of the continuity of nature. This effort also addresses the problem of identity of the same object throughout a multiplicity of awareness. The key to the transcendental function of C-W is an explication of the constituting transcendental ego.[8*] The reality of the world is the accomplishment of the synthetic intendings of consciousness. These in turn constitute the automatic and active syntheses of identification and unification.[28]

---

* The transcendental ego is universal subjectivity correlative with all objectivity. It is not of the world but integral with the world as its noncausal, nontemporal, and nonspatial foundation. Husserl describes it as infinite and eternal.[28]

Automatic Syntheses. The automatic synthesis of inner-time-consciousness is the foundation of the life-world *(Lebenswelt)* and is continuously being constituted. Husserl uses the term "horizon" to refer to the unfocused life-world. One essential structure of the life-world is that every object has a horizon, which is also constituted through the unity of intentions, retentions, and protentions of the transcendental ego.[8] Table 6–1 depicts the dynamic unity of this horizon, co-intended by the transcendental ego positioned in the "Now." Involvement of effort or thematizing by an individual human is not described of automatic syntheses. Accordingly, inner-time-consciousness is thereby given as nonspatial, nontemporal, and noncausal.[8] The world is given, nonetheless, through multiple modes of awareness.

TABLE 6–1. PHENOMENOLOGICAL PERSPECTIVE: MULTIPLE MODES OF AWARENESS AND EXAMPLES OF KNOWLEDGE DOMAINS

Modes of Awareness (Examples)	C-W Objects-as-Meant	Domains of Knowledge (Examples)
Judging	*	
Doubting	*	Personal
Believing	*	Social
Hoping	*	
Intuiting (intellectually)	*	Essences (identities) patterns
Remembering	*	
Imagining	*	
Conceptualizing	*	Spatial–temporal–causal as well as non-spatial–temporal–causal
Loving	*	
Valuing	*	
Anticipating	*	
Perceiving	*	
Hearing	*	
Seeing	*	Spatial–temporal–causal world
Touching	*	
Tasting	*	
Smelling	*	
Intuiting (sensibly)	*	Conditioned by space, time, and cause
Grieving	*	
Forgetting	*	
Avoiding	*	
Striving	*	Transcendental, mundane world
Pushing	*	
Pulling	*	
Hurting	*	
Resisting	*	

*Symbolic—any focus selected in nature or the created world.

Conversely, the world is not "created" by an individual but rather constituted automatically through the unity of dynamic intendings of inner-time-consciousness. Thus, C-W is changing and increasing in diversity and complexity through ongoing automatic and active syntheses.

The transcendental ego as the source of all types of intendings persists throughout the increasing complexity of the life-world while constituting as well as being constituted itself. In addition, the world is never separate from consciousness. Furthermore, reasoning is not yet described, but only its rudimentary tendings, which Husserl called the "doxic position" toward all objects, co-intended as actual.[28] In other words, the life-world is taken as "actual" even though it is given in the initial vague form to consciousness.

Synthesis of Identification. Synthesis of identification is another form of synthesis in inner-time-consciousness, again described first by Husserl's investigations. Synthesis of identification presupposes the life-world constituted by automatic synthesis, which constitutes the conditions for its possibility.[8] Synthesis of identities in its rudimentary form is not a function of reason yet, but is given as constituted by consciousness (C-W) as a passive activity fundamental to all other forms of identification. In other words, the world is given as a synthesized identity with its own unity, before reason and effort are involved actively. Furthermore, identification of relations between identities presupposes each identity given as its own.

Synthesis of identification Husserl submits is describable only after gaining access to inner-time-consciousness by performing the transcendental epoche and eidetic epoche (bracketing). Without their performance, the straightforward awareness of the world does not gain access to inner-time-consciousness of the world. Reflection on objects as intended "by me" is required. The world as co-intended, given nonspatially, nontemporally, and noncausally, is then accessible. Thus rendered accessible, the syntheses of identification automatically signify objects as identities co-intended by multiple modes of awareness. The objects as identities co-intended are seen against the horizon of fulfilled intentions of inner-time-consciousness.

Synthesis of Unification. Synthesis of unifications is also a type of synthesis described by Husserl. The primary writings were done with Eugene Fink between 1920 and 1930. However, these writings are not yet accessible to general scholars but are currently being interpreted and translated.[25]

In general, Husserl designates "synthesis" as a "systematic unity," which is a "primal form belonging to consciousness."[9] Synthesis is not a constructive operation like Kant's productive imagination. Berger further clarifies Husserl's description of synthesis through the phenomenological method and distinguishes it from "making" or even "remaking" anything; unity is "seen," not "constructed." Synthesis is "grasped by intuition."[3]

Synthesis is not to be taken as some kind of ego activity or function but rather designates the dynamic nature of the constituting C-W, which is identifiable as intuitive and creative.[3]

Transcendental Epoche and Eidos Epoche (Bracketing)

The most characteristic move advocated by Husserl for a transcendental phenomenology is a performance of the transcendental epoche and eidos epoche (bracketing). In brief, access to the constituting and constituted C-W requires a temporary setting aside of the familiar common-sense and scientific explanations of the world.

Transcendental Epoche

Husserl advocates the practice of avoiding premature judgments about the status of phenomena (object as intended) whereby the world is judged according to the conditions of space, time, and causality among other things.[4]

Eidos Epoche (Bracketing)

When we have performed the transcendental epoche, the structure of intentionality (inner-time-consciousness) is rendered accessible and intelligible. Most importantly, this epoche avoids making a distinction between what is actual (being) and what is possible (nonbeing). Since the actual world must first be possible but not all possible worlds must be actual, the actual world is less encompassing. The world of possibility is broader than the possibility for the conditions of knowledge represented by the categories of Kant, and is infinite but nonetheless effable (knowable). Accordingly, Husserlian phenomenologists consider all that is perceptible, conceivable, and imaginable on equal terms. Therefore, "real" and "unreal," "being" and "nonbeing" are distinctions that are not of concern within the transcendental phenomenological theory of knowledge. If objects are intended through any mode of awareness, whether through straightforward awareness or reflection, intellectual, essential, or sensible intuition, or imagination, the objects intended are "attended to" and tested as apodictic evidence by the Principle of All Principles (principle of phenomenological testing of all possible objectivity).

A major postulate of Husserl's epistemology is that transcendental subjectivity throughout multiple modes of awareness is the source of all objectivity.[8] Therefore, Husserl posits that the means to know all objects in the world is by a thoroughgoing investigation of consciousness of the world (C-W).

Multiple Modes of Awareness of C-W

The multiple modes of awareness are always described as integral with their object domain—as "object intended" in Cairns' term.[3] Central to the phenomenological perspective is the object identity, which obtains throughout the multiple modes of awareness. Table 6–1 illustrates two essential relations that obtain within the structure of C-W: (1) it illuminates the multiple modes of awareness by which all objects can be intended; (2) it places in perspective the varied ways modes of awareness have been delimited within the sciences. For example, the range of awareness modalities counted as valid in the positivist and logical positivist philosophy of science appears quite narrow in contrast to the broad range counted as apodictic evidence in phenomenology as a rigorous science of the life-world. Table 6–1 illustrates the relation that obtains between (1) the multiple modes of awareness, (2) the totality of all possible objectivity's (all objects in the world), and (3) the domains of knowledge that are accessible through the phenomenological perspective.

Table 6–1 exemplifies but does not exhaust the varied modalities of awareness possible to C-W in general. Many modalities are co-intendings with any number of the others, depending upon the nature of the object(s) intended. For example, access to any one or all objects is possible through one, many, or all of the modalities of awareness. A "train" is an object-intended that can be intuited (intellectually, sensibly, and essentially), imagined conceptually, sensibly, or concretely; judged, valued, remembered, anticipated, avoided, resisted as well as seen, heard, touched, and smelled. Upon reflection, these objects-intended are domains of knowledge whose co-intendings commonly occur together and are directed to the same kinds of objects.

Thus, the domains of knowledge identifiable include some of the following: meanings, essences, concepts, and constructs of time, space, and cause; concepts and constructs as nontemporal, nonspatial, noncausal; personal, social, intersubjective world as meant, mundane world unthematized, taken for granted. The modes of awareness are limited by Kant's categories of space, time, and causality as well as by Carnap's theory of physicalism in the positivist and logical-positivist philosophies of science. Thus, access to the world of objectivity is limited to the actual concrete world and/or as it is sensibly intuited, imagined, or conceived in terms of time, space, and cause. Moreover, the possible worlds beyond such modalities and conditions for knowledge are not accessible, therefore not intelligible in such a restricted view of objectivity.

In summary, the logical and intuitive insight gained through this explication tends to support the position for a broadened definition of experience as well as to "see" the integral relation of the knower and the known in the acquisition of all knowledge. The relevancy of Husserlian phenomenology to the multifaceted concerns of nursing in general is illuminated by this explication. It is the position of this thesis that, given the holistic concerns of nursing manifest through the majority of theories of nursing, the analyses of experience achieved through phenomenology renders it a congruent and desirable approach for nursing science. To strengthen this argument, a specific nursing conceptual framework was selected for analysis focusing on one of its major postulates.

CONGRUENCY OF HUSSERL'S "INTENTIONALITY" AND ROGERS' "FOUR-DIMENSIONALITY"

The exploration of congruency of Husserl's "principle of intentionality" (P-I) and of Rogers' postulate of "four-dimensionality" (4-D) assumes the central role each plays within its respective system. The Rogerian conceptual system is viewed as an ontology, stating a position about the nature of humans and the environment. Husserlian phenomenology as a rigorous science is viewed as an epistemology describing a theory of knowledge. An explication of congruency between the two is thus viewed in this study accordingly, as congruency between a holistic nursing conceptual system and an integral philosophy of science.

Points of congruence between P-I and 4-D are most evident in the following areas: (1) the point of departure for the authors' postulates; (2) the primary focus of the authors' postulates; (3) the universal nature of the postulates of 4-D and P-I; and (4) the ways of acquiring knowledge indicated by the nature of these postulates.

The Point of Departure for the Authors' Postulates

First of all, the point of departure for both Rogers and Husserl in positing their postulates is that of personal knowledge. For example, Rogers describes the world of man and environment "as she sees it," not on the authority of another's description of theory.[24] Likewise, Husserl describes consciousness of the world "as he sees it as originally given."[8] Both Rogers and Husserl suggest temporarily putting aside (not rejecting) the world view of Newtonian physics and natural sciences for the purpose of gaining another view that is more evidentially given. The "I" is the ultimate court of appeal for each of their postulates.

Husserl calls this originary evidence "apodictic evidence"; Rogers describes this kind of evidence as "the kind you must go and see for yourself."[24]

The Primary Focus of the Authors' Postulates

The primary focus of Rogers and Husserl is on generic (universal) human beings in the world. For instance, Rogers'[16, 17] focus is on generic unitary human beings. Husserl[8] likewise focuses on universal consciousness of the world. Neither of the authors' primary focus is on individual, particular human beings located in the world under certain conditions. This is true, for both authors' descriptions of the focus they postulate must be the starting point of their science. As the focal point, this universal is to be used as a gauge for all other knowledge acquired.

For both Rogers and Husserl, the object of their focus obtains a necessary integral view. That is, for Rogers, the term "unitary human beings" implies human beings always in mutual process with the environment. For Husserl, the term "consciousness of the world" means consciousness is always integral to the world. Neither can be known isolated from the other, and each requires the other. Thus, both Rogers and Husserl have an integral viewpoint–standpoint.

The Nature of the Postulates of 4-D and P-I

The following discussion is aided by reference to two figures given in this text: Figure 6–1, showing four-dimensionality,[17] and Figure 6–2, showing the principle of intentionality.[8] Also, the discussion is developed according to four major points of congruence: (1) positionality in the world, (2) identity and multiplicity, (3) view of causality in the world, and (4) nature of the known.

Positionality of Humans in the World

Rogers[17] sees the human field embedded in the environmental field as synonymous with the "Infinite Now" and as nontemporal in the sense of experiencing the past or future or present. "Infinite Now," however, implies, as she suggests, a time flowing. Likewise, Husserl describes the position of consciousness in the world as the "Infinite Now" of "inner-time-consciousness." Consciousness in the world is nontemporal in regard to "scientific time."[28]

In addition, both Rogers and Husserl describe universal humans in the world as nonspatial: in other words, not necessarily located in place or conditioned by particular concrete, physical attributes. Rogers indicates the unitary human being is an infinite being whose manifestations include "paranormal events" considered irrational otherwise in a three-dimensional world. The realm of infinite possibility as well as the actual is included by Rogers. Husserl's postulate of P-I also describes C-W as nonspatial, including the world of possibility, not only of actuality. Thus, not all realities are necessarily determined to be concretized.

Identity and Multiplicity

Rogers' and Husserl's postulates both indicate that in man's relation to the world, an identity is recognizable throughout diversity and change. For example, Rogers posits that the human field is identified by *pattern,* defined as that of unitary human beings, which is always integral, irreducible to parts. Also as positioned, the identity of unitary human beings is always the "Infinite Now" for any given individual. Identity as a unitary human being is not contradictory to multidimensional, innovative change and is continuously evolving.[18] Pattern, thus, is not static but dynamic, yet always its own identity.[23]

In similar ways, Husserl posits the essential structure of intentionality as the identity of the universal consciousness of the world. The identity of C-W is dynamic, "constituted" and "constituting" itself infinitely through the multiple modes of awareness. In both Rogers' and Husserl's postulates, then, identity is seen as manifesting diversity and dynamic activity. The one and the many are given in the same view as integral rather than contradictory. This leads to the discussion of a key premise regarding the nature of syntheses and the constitution of reality in C-W.

View of Causality

Rogers' 4-D indicates that the human field in mutual process with the environmental field is "noncausal." Furthermore, four-dimensional reality is perceived as "a nonlinear domain without spatial or temporal attributes."[21] Therefore, the type of synthesis implied by the pattern of unitary human beings is a nondeterministic type of synthesis. Neither the human field nor the environmental field is viewed in isolation or as causing the other.

Similarly, Husserl[8] posits universal intentionality as constituting itself and the world. "Constituting" is not a synthesis of parts into a whole, but rather a synthesis of identity and unity, which is first of all automatic and ongoing, without effort or accomplished by a particular reasoning and willing individual person. The universal synthesis of intentionality is ongoing and infinite through multiple modes of awareness of the world. Therefore, synthesis is never final or complete.

Though not explicit in Rogers, it can be implied that syntheses of individual unitary human beings furthermore manifest reason, creativity, understanding, and other diversities that indicate an evolution of pattern from the noncausal, nonlinear universal reality in the direction of greater complexity and possibility of human life in general.

Nature of the Known

Rogers' 4-D reality is perceived as a synthesis of nonlinear coordinates "from which innovative change continuously and evolutionally emerges."[18] Since Rogers states that the world she describes is the world "as she sees it," it can be implied that the nature of 4-D reality is reality as known by Rogers and others who share the same viewpoint.

Husserl's epistemology, based on the principle of intentionality, describes reality constituted by consciousness as always "progressive, infinite, and tentative" (transcendental in his view). Even though the totality of all objectivity is a goal of transcendental phenomenology, it is acknowledged as never achieved in totality. In addition, the task of phenomenology, as of all philosophy, is to define the limits of the possible, not the limits of the actual, concretized world. Therefore, knowledge of the world is never complete and final because there are always more possibilities that can affirm or falsify what is known. Husserl was called the "philosopher of infinite tasks" by Natanson,[10] which aptly describes the nature of his epistemology.

Ways of Acquiring Knowledge Indicated by the Authors' Postulates

The most difficult point on which to determine congruency between Husserl's P-I and Rogers' 4-D is in the ways these authors suggest knowledge is gained of universal humans in the world. Reasons for the difficulty are not necessarily a lack of the authors' references to this issue but rather the inconsistencies advocated within the writings of Rogers; specifically, the view put forth in Chapters 11, 12, 13, and 14 of her major text[16] in contrast to all of her other writings. This evidence warrants a study in itself. However, the points of congruency related to 4-D and P-I are the only ones addressed in this section.

Of major importance is the evidence that Rogers[22] advocates a type of synthesis, one that does not predict knowledge of the whole from knowledge of the parts. This indicates that the kind of synthesis advocated by Kant in the notion of "productive imagination" and "a priori synthetic judgments" is not the kind meant by Rogers. Instead, the synthesis described by Husserl, which is noncausal, nonlinear, and automatic in nature, is congruent with Rogers' synthesis. As such, Husserl's synthesis begins with integral evidence constituted by C-W. Most uniquely, Husserl sees consciousness as the only access to knowledge of all objectivity and as inseparable. Rogers'[18] focus, unitary human being, is also advocated as the way, through personal knowledge; that is, by individual, thinking, feeling, sensing unitary human beings. For both Rogers and Husserl the reality spoken of as known is the effable world integral with the knowing unitary human being. For example, Rogers advocates ways of pushing back the frontiers of knowledge, and Husserl advocates performing the transcendental epoche and epidetic epoche. Specifically, Rogers suggests moving away from the familiar view of the world based on Newtonian physics. She invites one to move from solely viewing humans as particular, temporally–spatially located individuals in a causal world toward viewing humans as generic, universal realities.

Both Rogers and Husserl indicate that there are multiple ways required in the development of a self-given, personal-knowledge foundation for understanding universal humans in the world. Rogers[18, 20] states that a 4-D view of unitary human beings requires considerable abstract thinking, imagination, and imaginative synthesis as well as contemplation on principles. She uses analogy, poetry and illustrations, and readings on lateral thinking as opposed to vertical thinking to clear away obstacles for the possibility of "ahas" (creative insights).

Husserl advocates the transcendental epoche and eidetic epoche to temporarily set aside the spatial–temporal–causal world of natural science and Newtonian physics and any judgments of questions about the being or nonbeing of objects as intended. Rather, take as meant the world given through the multiple modes of awareness, and consider the limits of all possibilites of objects, not only the limits of the actual, concrete world.

Both Husserl and Rogers regard this move as necessary to gain access to the awareness of the universal identity and diversity of integral humans in the world. Just as significant, both Husserl and Rogers indicate simple observation is not enough, but rather multiple modes of awareness are used to view unitary human beings in all possible ways. To gain access to (really see) the universal nature of humans in the world, contemplation is suggested by Rogers, and reflection is imperative for Husserl. In fact, Husserl's emphasis is called "the radical reduction" or, better translated, "the radical unbuilding" for the possibility of knowledge from the founding principle of intentionality.[28]

CONCLUSIONS

Two conclusions can be drawn about the nature of knowledge posited from this philosophical analysis: (1) The nature of knowledge of unitary human beings described by four-dimensionality requires a philosophy of science that defines human experience of phenomena in the broadest possible way. (2) In accordance with the first conclusion, a science of humans in the world requires a theory of knowledge (epistemology) in which the knower and the known are integral, as opposed to being viewed as separate, and viewed as equal in mutual involvement, as opposed to being determined by either one isolated from the other. These conclusions are relevant particularly for the development of a conceptual system of any kind for reasons related to levels of knowledge.

IMPLICATIONS

The basic question addressed by this philosophical inquiry[11] asks whether an incongruity exists between a holistic nursing conceptual system (Rogers) and the philosophies of science advocated for the development and testing of knowledge.

Given the congruency between Husserlian phenomenology and the Rogerian conceptual system, a sound, convincing rationale is established for the use of this philosophy of science as an alternative for basic theoretical studies in Rogerian nursing science.

The major points of congruency with Husserlian phenomenology are the same points of incongruency with the prevailing logical positivist philosophy of science. Specifically, the postulate of Rogers' "four-dimensionality" is congruent with Husserl's "principle of intentionality" and incongruent with Carnap's theory of physicalism undergirding the logical positivist's principle of verification, which is the prevailing view of science in the twentieth century.

Nursing research in general requires a broader range of human experience than sensory experience (whether intuitive or perceptive) in the development and testing of conceptual systems, and for gaining better access to multifaceted human phenomena.

A tracing of the "idea of experience" from Descartes to twentieth-century philosophy of science outlines the limits and strengths of logical positivism, and indicates that Husserlian phenomenology as a rigorous science provides just such an experience. The broader range of experience is described as "multiple modes of awareness of all possible objectivities." These include "objects as meant" such as objects intuited, as imagined, as grieved, as perceived, as judged, as resisted, as believed, as conceived, as remembered, as forgotten, as lived, as anticipated, as expected, as forgiven, as held, as hoped, as well as sense-perceptible things.

RECOMMENDATIONS FOR FURTHER STUDY

The relevancy and potential benefit of Husserlian phenomenology for a helping profession have been illustrated, using one conceptual system in nursing (Rogers) as an example. However, the general applicability of the phenomenological perspective (analysis of experience), which is multifaceted and broad in scope, can now be illustrated through other basic research studies. In this way, the congruence or noncongruence of phenomenology as a rigorous science can be tested for relevancy to advance nursing theories with various phenomena of interest.

Comparative studies of the same phenomenon of concern from different perspectives are warranted in nursing's efforts to gain the most inclusive access possible to the phenomenon. The benefits from use of the phenomenological perspective and approach can be compared with those obtained through one or all of the following approaches: logical-positivist, ethnoscientific, historical, philosophical, positivist, esthetic, ethical, pragmatic, or existential.

Alternative approaches to nursing's phenomena require an analysis of the conditions for the possibility of knowledge and service. Both philosophical inquiry and phenomenology may provide the (conceptual) tools to meet these needs by gaining access to and clarifying the central phenomena of nursing education, research, and practice.

REFERENCES

1. Abbott EA: Flatland. New York, Dover, 1952
2. Berger G: The Cogito in Husserl's Philosophy. McLaughlin K (trans). Evanston, Ill, Northwestern University Press, 1972 (originally published 1941)
3. Cairns D: An approach to Husserlian phenomenology. In Kersten F, Zaner RM (eds): Criticisms and Continuation: Essays in Honor of Dorian Cairns. The Hague, Nijhoff, 1972
4. Carnap R: Psychology in physical language. Schick G (trans). In Ayer AJ (ed): Logical Positivism. New York, Free Press, 1959
5. Einstein A, et al.: The Principle of Relativity. New York, Dover, 1923
6. Gurwitsch A: Phenomenology and the Theory of Science. Embree L (ed). Evanston, Ill, Northwestern University Press, 1974
7. Hacking I (ed): Scientific Revolutions. Oxford Readings in Philosophy. London, Oxford University Press, 1981
8. Husserl E: Cartesian Meditations. Cairns, D (trans). The Hauge, Nijhoff, 1960 (Originally published 1933)
9. Husserl E: The Crisis of European Sciences. Carr D (trans). Evanston, Ill, Northwestern University Press, 1970 (Originally published 1934)
10. Natanson MA: Edmund Husserl: Philosopher of Infinite Tasks. Evanston, Ill, Northwestern University Press, 1973
11. Reeder F: Nursing Research, Holism, and Philosophies of Science: Points of Congruence Between M. E. Rogers and E. Husserl, doctoral dissertation. New York University 1984 (University Microfilms No. 84–21, 466)
12. Rogers ME: Educational Revolution in Nursing. New York, Macmillan, 1961
13. Rogers ME: Some comments on the theoretical basis of nursing practice. Nurs Sci 1:11, 1963
14. Rogers ME: Editorial. Nurs Sci 2:378–380, 1964
15. Rogers ME: Reveille in Nursing. Philadelphia, F. A. Davis, 1964
16. Rogers ME: Nursing science, research and researchers. In Teachers College Report. New York, Teachers College, 1967
17. Rogers ME: An Introduction to the Theoretical Basis of Nursing. Philadelphia, F. A. Davis, 1970
18. Rogers ME: Nursing: A science of unitary man. New York University, 1979 (unpublished)
19. Rogers ME: Nursing: A science of unitary man. In Reihl JP, Roy C (eds): Conceptual Models for Nursing Practice. New York, Appleton-Century-Crofts, 1980
20. Rogers ME: Science of unitary man: A paradigm for nursing. In Laskar GE (ed): Applied Systems of Cybernetics, Vol 4. Elmsford, NY, Pergamon Press, 1981

21. Rogers ME: Beyond the horizon. In Chaska N (ed): The Nursing Profession: A Time to Speak. New York, McGraw-Hill, 1982

22. Rogers ME: Nursing science: A science of unitary human beings: Glossary. New York University, 1983 (unpublished)

23. Rogers ME: Personal communication, 1983

24. Rogers ME: Science of unitary human beings: A paradigm for nursing. In Clements IW, Roberts FB (eds): Family Health: A Theoretical Approach. New York, Wiley, 1983

25. Sarter BJ: Interview with M. E. Rogers. New York University, 1983 (unpublished)

26. Spiegelberg H: The Pnenomenological Movement, 3rd ed. The Hague, Martinhoff, 1982 (Originally published 1965)

27. Thayer H: Meaning and Action—A Critical History of Pragmatism. New York, Bobbs-Merrill, 1968

28. Wiggins O: Senior seminar in Cartesian meditations, Edmund Husserl. Graduate Faculty, New School for Social Research, 1983 (unpublished papers)

7

The Science of Unitary Human Beings: Theoretical Issues, Methodological Challenges, and Research Realities

W. Richard Cowling, III

Nursing has the opportunity to develop a scientific base for practice that transcends the failures of the reductionistic and mechanistic perspective inherent in the biomedical model. The explication and testing of theory evolving from the Science of Unitary Human Beings proposed by Rogers is one clear path available for nursing to actualize this opportunity.[24, 26] The purpose of this chapter is to address crucial theoretical issues and methodological challenges that comprise the research realities of testing theory derived from the Science of Unitary Human Beings. The content was developed following the completion of such a theory-testing venture (Chapter 12) and reflects a perspective that has evolved as a consequence. The chapter is intended to address issues facing the researcher and is not meant as a criticism of past endeavors.

SIGNIFICANCE OF THE SCIENCE OF UNITARY HUMAN BEINGS

The significance of Rogers' conceptual system is that it gives nursing a clearly unique focus: the phenomenon of the unitary human being. "No other science or learned professional field deals with unitary man as a synergistic phenomenon whose behaviors cannot be predicted by knowledge of the parts."[26] Nursing can thus be contrasted to such disciplines as psychology, which emphasizes the person as a psychological phenomenon, or sociology, which emphasizes the sociological context of the person. The Science of Unitary Human Beings gives nursing a distinct identity.

Further, the Science of Unitary Human Beings offers a bold contrast to the predominant biomedical model, which is firmly grounded in Cartesian ideology, postulating a strict separation of mind and body with the body viewed as an intricate machine.[6] According to the biomedical model, like any other machine, the body can be understood in terms of the arrangement and functioning of the parts. Consequently, biomedical research aims at understanding the human by the method of reduction. The failure of this reductionistic approach to health care was recently highlighted by Capra, who noted the following points:[6] It has resulted in the split of health care practices into the medical and psychiatric realms, leaving the understanding of human phenomena fragmented; the philosophical and existential issues surrounding illness are avoided; emphasis has been placed upon an engineering approach to health, with the major strategies being technological in nature; the effects of misused technology include increased health care costs, iatrogenic illness, and generalized dehumanization of the hospital setting. In general, attention of the medical profession is upon disease rather than the whole person.

In addition, the Science of Unitary Human Beings is significantly different from other nursing frameworks. Barrett distinguishes two types of nursing conceptual frameworks based upon whether nursing knowledge is viewed as evolution or revolution.[2] Evolutionary nursing frameworks are consistent with a view of nursing science as a synthesis of knowledge from other disciplines uniquely utilized by nursing. Evolutionary conceptual frameworks, like the biomedical model, describe the human being as a synthesis or integration of parts. In contrast, according to Barrett, the Science of Unitary Human Beings can be categorized as revolutionary because "rather than end with synthesis, it begins with a unique synthesis which constitutes the creation of a new product."[2] Newman[19] has also noted that beginning with the whole is the crucial difference in the Science of Unitary Human Beings.

It can also be argued that the Science of Unitary Human Beings provides a framework for nursing that shows remarkable consistency with concepts emerging in a new world view of reality.[6, 11] Just as Newtonian physics serves as the basis for the reductionistic and mechanistic world view, the conceptual revolutions in physics, rooted in the work of Einstein, serve as the basis for a new world view termed holistic and ecological.[5, 6, 29, 34] The new world view provides increased potential for understanding health in the context of the whole person. It also offers explanatory concepts for previously unexplained phenomena and therapeutic modalities. The concepts delineated by Rogers[24, 26] in the Science of Unitary Human Beings—energy fields, openness, pattern, four-dimensionality—as well as the principles of homeodynamics, are consistent with concepts in the new physics and the accompanying world view (see Chapter 3). While it is clear that the Science of Unitary Human Beings' perspective articulates with the emerging world view of reality, it is important to note that nowhere is Rogers' framework duplicated.[2]

The significance of a unique nursing conceptual framework should not be underestimated. Fawcett[9] linked the emergence of nursing as a separate discipline and independent profession to the identification of a distinct body of knowledge about phenomena central to nursing. Rogers[26] correlated the explication of nursing's knowledge base to the transition of nursing from prescience to science. While views seem to differ on which framework is best for nursing and on ways to derive theory, there seems to be no apparent disagreement among nursing scholars on the need for theoretical knowledge and the role of research in testing theory.

The Science of Unitary Human Beings has rich potential for directing research that will provide a substantial base of knowledge for nursing. It has provided the foundations for several research endeavors (see Chapters 8 to 15);[12] others are in progress, and still others have been proposed.[17, 21] Conceptual and methodological issues need to be addressed by the researcher whose aim is to generate studies from the Rogerian unitary conceptual system.

CONCEPTUAL AND METHODOLOGICAL ISSUES

Critical elements of the research process that are especially problematic for researchers utilizing the Rogerian perspective include: (1) theory postulation represented in the hypothesis statement; (2) identification of variables; (3) operationalization and measurement of variables; and (4) selection of a research design. While these elements present distinctive concerns for the researcher, they are interrelated components of the process.

Theory Derivation

The first crucial step in the research process is the derivation of a testable theory evolving from the conceptual system. The logic utilized to derive the theorem should be consistent with the basic premises of the system. As Kim[15] has noted, Rogers' basic premises explaining relationships and characteristics of human and environmental fields are evolution and noncausality. In addition, Rogers embraces the premise of open, negentropic, irreducible energy fields.

Logic that does not fragment, separate, or isolate aspects of the unitary human beings is requisite for deriving theoretically sound hypothesis statements congruent with the Rogerian conceptual system. For example, Newman has noted that a major difficulty with the scientific method is its tendency to be context-stripping when used for context-dependent phenomena, such as human experience.[20] The testing of theory from the Science of Unitary Human Beings requires that theorems be logically consistent with the contextual features of human energy fields and their developmental process. The contextual features are articulated in the premises of the conceptual system.

An example from my experience is the derivation of a theorem from the principle of helicy, which specifies that unitary human development is characterized by an increasing complexity and diversity of a continuously innovative, nonrepetitive field wave pattern[26] (see Chapter 12). I contended that, inherent in an open system of complex fields, innovation of field pattern emerges out of diversity of field pattern. Diversity and innovation are mutual pattern characteristics that should correlate, according to the principle of helicy. The greater the degree of diversity, the greater the innovation of the pattern. Thus, the main theoretical proposition was that a positive relationship exists between the field pattern characteristics of diversity and innovativeness.[8]

Similarly, Raile-Alligood (see Chapter 13) utilized the logic that if the nature of developmental change were helical, one could expect human field pattern manifestations of the helical process in human individuals.[23] From the principle of helicy, these pattern manifestations were proposed to correlate positively. Ference (see Chapter 9) derived the theorem that there is an empirical relationship among correlates of unitary human development from the principle of resonancy.[10] Her logic was to connect constructs to the empirical world through rules of correspondence.

Ference addressed a chief concern in the researcher's logical construction for deriving testable theorems: Is it particulate to isolate variables postulated in the direction of change, not examining completely the synergistic nature of human development?[10] This question reflects the concern of being reductionistic in one's approach and poses a major dilemma.

Examination of theoretical development in nursing reveals a tendency to advocate reductionism as an approach to understanding humans.[33] Recently Kim has advocated a typology for theoretical analysis "as a tool and guide that can be used to separate out aspects of the real world we encounter into coherent sets of theoretical elements."[16] Walker and Avant advocate three approaches to theory construction: analysis, synthesis, and derivation.[31] Analysis is described as dissecting a whole into its component parts to increase understanding. Synthesis involves combining pieces of information that may have theoretical connections. Derivation is characterized as using analogy or metaphors to transpose and redefine concepts from one context to another. If the function of conceptual systems in nursing is to focus our thinking in a particular way, as has been suggested by Newman,[19] Rogers' conceptual system would direct us to new ways of theoretical thinking more compatible with its underlying assumptions.

Derivation of theory from Rogers' conceptual system requires a new way of thinking beyond our traditional logic that does not accommodate the basic assumptions of the unitary stance, namely:

1. Irreducibility of the human to parts
2. Noncausality
3. Continual change

Three modes of thinking that embrace each of these assumptions are:

1. Existentialism
2. Ecological thinking
3. Dialectical thinking

These modes offer possible viable alternatives to the analytic mode of thinking, which is basically one of reduction.

Existentialism as a way of thinking accommodates irreducibility to parts, which essentially places a focus on a wide information source rather than on a very narrow one. It can best be explained in relation to two other more traditional modes of thinking: rationalism and pragmatism.[27]

Rationalism begins with a generalization of a concept. Steps in the process include: (1) defining terms; (2) stating assumptions; (3) drawing conclusions based on assumptions; and (4) predicting from temporal sequencing. Reason and Rowan have noted that rationalism is most generally applicable to situations where rigor is possible.[27] Thus it is applicable primarily to closed tautological systems where all relevant information is available and where the logic of the situation is well known. Examples of such systems given by Reason and Rowan include geometries, number systems, and closed sets.

Pragmatism is a method characterized as "recurrent formulation, deduction, test in reality, detection of difference between expectation and findings, and feeding back the error into the formulation until the difference between the new expectation and the latest look at reality becomes arbitrarily small."[13] Pragmatism is viewed as an appropriate response in situations where there is more information than can be handled rationally, but where experimentation is possible due to the expectation of convergence of results. Technology and most of the physical sciences are appropriate areas relevant for pragmatism as a mode of thinking.

Existentialism becomes an appropriate mode of inquiry when the amount of information increases so that experimentation is no longer possible with any assurance of convergence.[27] Existentialism is described by Hainer as beginning with experience, phenomena, and existence as they are perceived. "Concepts arise out of the uniquely human process of perceiving, pattern (Gestalt) forming, of symbolising, of comparing, and of conceptualising, which are not explicitly conscious."[13] Existentialism is also described as a contemplative, relaxed approach that allows values, meaning, and alternatives to suggest themselves through free association and metaphor.[4]

Contrasted with rationalism and pragmatism, existentialism is a state of consciousness in which information is processed in a different mode.[27] Rationalism leads to propositional knowledge, pragmatism to propositional or practical knowledge, and existentialism to propositional, practical, or experiential knowledge. Existentialism provides an alternative approach to theory construction that is logically congruent with Rogers' system.

Ecological thinking is an alternative form of logic that has potential usefulness in theory construction because it accommodates the premise of noncausality. This mode of thinking, which derives from cybernetics and systems theory, includes the notion of patterning as a replacement for cause and effect. However, it falls short in other areas that encompass ideas of feedback and redundancy incompatible with the unitary human perspective. Bateson has employed ecological thinking in his work entitled *Mind and Nature*.[3] Ecological thinking represents an epistemological shift that has consequences for theory and research from the Rogerian perspective.

Dialectical thinking provides a way of addressing the continuity of change because it places all the emphasis upon change. "Instead of talking about static structures, it talks about process and movement."[27] In other words, it is in line with philosophies that are less concerned with what is, such as the diagnostic perspective, in which we "label it and fix it;" rather, dialectical thinking lets us look at how it changes. Wilson and Fitzpatrick have recently detailed the compatibility of dialectical thinking with Rogers' perspective.[33]

One potential answer to the dilemma created by the reductionism of the scientific method may be the way in which we conceptualize the phenomena under investigation. For the investigator utilizing Rogers' framework, human behavior can be conceptualized as a manifestation of the human field pattern reflecting its qualities or characteristics. Human behavior provides information about the human field pattern but is not the human field itself. There is a distinctive difference in viewing behavior as a manifestation of the whole rather than as a component of the whole. The theorem, as reflected in the hypothesis statement, links various manifestations of the field pattern, placing them in context of the whole.

Selection of Variables

The next crucial problem area addressed is selection of variables that reflect unitary human development. The researcher may employ several methods to arrive at variables that have meaning within this particular framework. A major consideration in selecting variables for study within the Science of Unitary Human Beings is conceptual congruence with the system.

One approach to arriving at variables is reviewing correlates proposed by Rogers (see Chapter 2) that serve as descriptors of unitary human development.[25] The terminology used to describe relative changes in the development process includes *timeless, transcendent, ethereal, beyond waking,* and *visionary.* In addition, unitary human development is viewed as moving from less differentiation to more differentiation. After reviewing these correlates, I selected the variables of mystical experience and differentiation to capture the human field pattern characteristic of diversity. The nature of unitary human development is also innovative, as manifested in the correlate of imaginativeness. Because imaginativeness is implied in the creative process, creativity was chosen as another variable.

A principal criticism of selection of variables from other frameworks is that they are therefore incompatible because of different assumptions. In two studies derived from the Science of Unitary Human Beings, the variable of differentiation was chosen as a correlate of development.[8, 10] While this variable has been the focus of intensive, long-term study within the field of psychology, the concept is rather universally defined regardless of the theoretical framework—that is, increasing complexity, diversity, and heterogeneity as reflected in the negentropic process of unitary human development.

One way to identify appropriate variables from non-Rogerian frameworks is previous research linking variables that are conceptually consistent with the Science of Unitary Human Beings. There is a tendency to neglect studies linking variables based on other frameworks. The Rogerian conceptual system may provide an alternative explanation for relationships among variables or explain those that are not accounted for by the particular framework.

Another approach to variable selection involves the organization of several variables into a set that attempts to capture a wider array of pattern properties. For example, the pattern characteristic of diversity was identified by differentiation and mystical experience in my study because they comprised a more complete set than either variable alone. Accepting the common definition of diversity as having differing forms of qualities, the two variables were viewed as representing a number of potential differing forms or qualities within a pattern profile.

The final approach, which is less laden with conceptual problems, is the elaboration of a variable reflecting a construct of the conceptual system. Ference's work is an example of such an approach, which involved the development of the construct as well as instrumentation to measure the variable of human field motion. Human field motion was defined as "experiential, multidimensional position of the human energy field pattern."[10] The major disadvantages of this approach are the time involved in pilot study and the reliabilty and validity of questions raised. However, the potential for conceptual validity is greater than in utilizing variables derived from other frameworks.

Operationalization and Measurement of Variables

Another prime consideration of the adequacy of research is operationalization and measurement of proposed research variables. The ideal situation is the development of instrumentation. Barrett suggested the need for "retooling to capture theoretically proposed manifestations."[2] As noted earlier, this approach offers the greatest potential for construct validity of measures of unitary human phenomena.

It is important to note that the measurement process always deals with abstractions. The researcher is measuring attributes or characteristics of an object, and not the object itself. Measurement procedures constitute the operational definitions of concepts, and concepts cannot be adequately measured until the nature of them is fully specified.[22]

These principles of measurement have implications for study within the unitary framework. The human energy field is an abstraction utilized to capture the phenomenon of interest. It is a conceptualization that is further specified by attributes of openness, four-dimensionality, negentropy, and pattern. Further specification of the human field includes the attributes of diversity, innovation, complexity, and nonrepetitive rhythmicities. Even further specification of attributes are the developmental correlates, which are behavioral manifestations of the unitary human field proposed by Rogers.

The correlates provide a link to appropriate operationalization and measurement decisions. Central to these decisions should be a constant concern for adhering to the basic assumptions of the conceptual system that identify its uniqueness: (1) the synergistic nature of the unitary human being, (2) the nonlinear, noncausal, probabilistic nature of change, and (3) the relativity of change, varying continuously within and between human fields.[25]

The ideal of measurement in the current scientific method is one that results in a quantitative score. However, in the Rogerian framework, the ideal may be very different. Barrett stated that "to capture what happens in the field beyond what an observer can perceive through the senses requires appropriate tools that measure the nonmaterial, contemplative, direct experiencing features of unitary man in terms of qualities as well as quantities."[2] Similarly, Capra proposed a shift in conceptualizing science toward a focus on qualities rather than quantities having a basis in shared experience rather than verifiable measurements.[6] The data for such a science would consist of experience, subjective to varying degrees, which cannot be quantified or analyzed into fundamental units. Such approaches are necessary in order to transcend the reductionism of current scientific methodology.

Selecting measures of proposed variables is a crucial decision that determines how meaningful research will be within the originating conceptual system. Subjective, self-report measures and those based upon an experiential, phenomenological perspective may be methodologically more compatible to the study of variables within the Science of Unitary Human Beings. Such measures allow for capturing the experiential features manifested by the human energy field. Ellis, as reported by Newman, suggested, "the human being is the best instrument to assess human experience."[20] Consequently, self-descriptive measures may be valid as indices of human field pattern characteristics. An example of this is the selection by two previous researchers of self-report instrumentation for measurement of creativity, rather than task- or function-oriented measures. Similarly, I chose a measure based on experiential phenomenological perspective for mystical experience.

Although it is not within the scope of this paper to discuss the problem of verification of truth claims, this problem is at the heart of criticism of study within the unitary framework. Wilber pointed out that, while there exist realms of data available to us, traditional science accepts as proof only that which is sensory in the form of physical data.[32] Further, he addressed the need for science to connect knowledge to experience in the broadest sense of direct apprehension: immediate givenness and intuition—sensory, mental, spiritual—and noted that *Geist* sciences, signifying those that encompass all realms of knowledge (not merely physical or empirical), rest on the relation of lived experience, expression, and understanding.

Wilber's conceptualization of realms of data may provide a significant step in broadening the research perspective in nursing.[31] Although his approach to realms of knowledge is somewhat hierarchical, it is not reductionistic. Understanding of the human is grasped through its external expressions. However, Wilber noted concisely,

> [t]he point is that the higher realms everywhere leave their footprints in the lower. The higher realms form and inform, create and mold, produce and alter, all manner of forms in the lower realms. But those productions cannot be grasped by the lower realms nor reduced to them.[32]

Using an analogy proposed by Wilber, we can say that attempting to verify unitary human phenomena in physical data such as brain physiology or blood pressure readings "is about as useful as hooking Einstein to an EEG in order to find out if E really does equal mc[2]."[32]

One of the major contributions of the Science of Unitary Human Beings is that it is inclusive rather than exclusive in recognizing data as a source of knowledge. While nursing's attempt to gain status as a professional discipline included embracing the scientific method, one of its repercussions was the exclusion of relevant data outside the sensory–physical realm. The Science of Unitary Human Beings has brought nursing back to an inclusive approach to knowledge, thus increasing the potential for a broader understanding of human experience.

Selecting a Research Design

Selecting a research design for a study derived from the Rogerian system is problematic because the design field is focused around the concept of causal relationships. The research design is judged in terms of its capacity to reveal causal relationships. If placed on a continuum, true experimental designs would be considered strongest and descriptive weakest.[22] Because the unitary system is a noncausal model of reality, strict experimental designs have questionable value for the purposes of research. However, experimental designs may be appropriate to specific theoretical propositions because they provide a mechanism for testing probabilistic change manifested from human–environmental process. Cook notes that quasiexperimentation grew from the realization, as genetics and particle physics advanced, that the world is probabilistically ordered in its essence.[7] An example of utilizing experimental or quasiexperimental designs within a Rogerian context would be the monitoring of indices of human field patterning in relation to introduced environmental change.

Designs that generate descriptive knowledge and explanatory knowledge are relevant because of the current level of theory development in the Science of Unitary Human Beings. Examples of such research designs include various descriptive correlational designs aimed at exploring the relationship between variables that are suggestive of unitary human field pattern characteristics. The intent of these studies is not to establish causal connections between variables. A correlation represents a relationship defined, interestingly, by Walizer and Wiener as "patterned mutual change."[30] The correlational design can provide evidence of patterned mutual change among variables that are proposed indices of the human field. Multivariate analysis procedures, particularly canonical correlation, can be useful methods for generating a constellation of variables representing human field pattern properties.

Other potential research approaches appropriate to the Rogerian framework that have been suggested include historical and philosophical.[2] Historical research may have value in highlighting historical evidence of the nature and direction of human and environmental change. Philosophical studies may contribute to the further specification of the conceptual entities as well as illuminate unitary phenomena. In addition, phenomenology may provide a means to address the qualitative, experiential features associated with unitary human change.

Survey research, often devalued as a scientific approach, would be appropriate in documenting potential evidence supporting a theory of increasing diversity as manifest in accelerating evolution. The uniqueness of each human energy field and the relative nature of change make the use of the case study or single case designs a rational approach to scientific inquiry. Finally, there is an essential need for methodological studies aimed at development, validation, and evaluation research tools and strategies for the unitary science framework.

METHODS

Some specific methods, which are described elsewhere as morphogenic or ideographic, imply a consideration for the uniqueness of the subject versus dealing with general dimensions of all subjects. Such methods encompass consultation with the richest of all sources of data concerning unitary development, namely, self-knowledge.

Some examples of morphogenic methods follow:

1. Matching is a method that suggests a fitting together of various records of personal expression in one subject. It has potential for the discovery of the degree to which a perceptible form quality saturates separate performances. The focus is on understanding and portraying the form that exists within human actions and that is not perceptible by focusing on individual pieces of behavior. Such a method could be useful in identifying correlates of unitary patterning for individuals.

2. Personal structural analysis was devised by Baldwin to focus on one woman through review of a long series of personal letters.[1] The object of interest was her unique thought structure. Again, emphasis is on unique individual pattern rather than parts. The object of interest could be redefined to focus on correlates of unitary development for those interested in investigating unitary patterning.

3. Shapiro also developed a morphogenic method that could be considered by the Rogerian researcher.[27] A questionnaire is constructed, based on extensive contact with one individual. The questionnaire is standard for this individual only and not relevant to others. It can be administered over a period of time to monitor development. This technique would be useful for the researcher interested in unitary development because it could focus upon the unique qualities of diverse and innovative field patterning for that individual.

4. Another morphogenic technique that could have applicability for the unitary perspective is to trace themes or intentions in a person's life. This information would be a useful index of field pattern.

5. Direct questioning is another potentially useful technique for the unitary perspective. Questions could be derived to focus upon individual patterning. Some examples of questions are, ''What experiences give you a feeling of completeness or fully functioning?'' ''What are your peak experiences?'' Projective methods and direct questioning could be combined for a more complete index of unitary patterning.

   The self-anchoring scale devised by Kirkpatrick and Cantril is an example of a more precise form of direct questioning.[14, 27] The technique is comprised of a simple diagram of a ladder with 10 rungs. Subjects are asked to describe in their own terms the best or ideal way of life. After being told that the top of the ladder represents their view of the ideal, they are asked to point to the rung that represents where they are to date, in the past, or where they will be in the future. Similarly, this technique might be used to investigate unitary change.

6. Another viable option is the Q-sort, which allows the subject to sort statements according to bipolar dimensions. Correlates of development could be approached using such a technique.

7. Imagery is another potentially useful method for the unitary perspective because it can be employed to transcend the linear logic of language. Images may provide a rich source of data for assessing the unitary field.

SUMMARY

The recent call for healthy debates about the adequacy of theoretical interpretations of the Rogerian conceptual system as used in research is valid.[15] It is also crucial that researchers utilizing the Rogerian system form networks that will facilitate open dialogue and shared knowledge. Research must proceed on several fronts, including focus on the relationship of human and environmental fields, description and specification of variables indicative of human field pattern properties, and methodological research. The explication of nursing's scientific base requires a ''stream'' of research rather than disconnected ''puddles.''

Research must continue within the traditional scientific context, if for no other reason than the pragmatics of acceptability for funding and general support. At the same time, we must all engage in the scholarly critique of existing scientific method of empiricism and the underlying philosophical tenets of reductionism with the aim of generating methodologies compatible with the unitary perspective proposed by Rogers.

Prominent scholars within and outside the discipline of nursing have challenged the reductionism of the empirical method. Some have even proposed entirely new alternative approaches to the discovery of knowledge, namely Capra, LeShan, Margenau, Newman, and Wilber.[5, 6, 18, 20, 32] The relevance of research within the Science of Unitary Human Beings perspective is heralded by the failures of the old world perspective. LeShan and Margenau have rightly noted that we must find a new way to view reality or ''go under.''[8]

Clearly, the Science of Unitary Human Beings provides a new way of organizing knowledge and of conceptualizing reality that distinguishes it from other perspectives. Creative research endeavors that are conceptually congruent with its premises will contribute to the explication of a scientific base for nursing practice that addresses the full potential of unitary human beings.

REFERENCES

1. Baldwin AL: Personal structural analysis: A statistical method for investigation of the single personality. J Abnorm Soc Psych 37:163–183, 1942
2. Barrett EA: Nursing conceptual frameworks as bases for research. Paper presented at Upsilon Chapter, Sigma Theta Tau Research Conference, New York University, New York, Nov 1980
3. Bateson G: Mind and Nature: A Necessary Unity. New York, Dutton, 1979
4. Borton T: Reach, Touch and Teach. New York, McGraw-Hill, 1970
5. Capra F: The Tao of Physics. Berkeley, Shambhala, 1975
6. Capra F: The Turning Point: Science, Society and the Rising Culture. New York, Simon & Schuster, 1982
7. Cook TD: Quasi-experimentation: Its ontology, epistemology, and methodology. In Morgan G (ed): Beyond Method: Strategies for Social Research. Beverly Hills, Sage, 1983, pp 74–94
8. Cowling WR: The Relationship of Mystical Experience, Differentiation, and Creativity in College Students: An Empirical Investigation of the Principle of Helicy in Rogers' Science of Unitary Man, doctoral dissertation. New York University, 1983 (University Microfilms Publication No. 84–06, 283)
9. Fawcett J: A declaration of nursing independence: The relation of theory and research to nursing practice. J Nurs 10:36–39, 1980
10. Ference HM: The Relationship of Time Experience, Creativity Traits, Differentiation, and Human Field Motion: An Empirical Investigation of Rogers' Correlates of Synergistic Human Development, doctoral dissertation. New York University, 1979 (University Microfilms)
11. Ferguson M: The Aquarian Conspiracy: Personal and Social Transformation in the 1980's. Los Angeles, J. P. Tarcher, 1980
12. Floyd JA: Research using Rogers's conceptual system: Development of a testable theorem. Adv Nurs Sci 5:37–48, 1983
13. Hainer R: Rationalism, pragmatism, and existentialism: Perceived but undiscovered multi-cultural problems. In Glatt E, Shelly MS (eds): The Research Society. New York, Gordon & Breach, 1968, pp. 7–50
14. Kilpatrick FP, Cantril H: Self-anchoring scale: A measure of the individual's unique reality world. J Individ Psychol 16:158–170, 1960
15. Kim HS: Use of Rogers's conceptual system in research: Comments. Nurs Res 32:89–91, 1983
16. Kim HS: The Nature of Theoretical Thinking in Nursing. E. Norwalk, Conn, Appleton-Century-Crofts, 1983
17. Krieger D: Foundations for Holistic Health Nursing Practices; The Renaissance Nurse. Philadelphia, Lippincott, 1981
18. LeShan L, Margenau H: Einstein's Space and Van Gogh's Sky: Physical Reality and Beyond. New York, Macmillan, 1982

19. Newman M: Theory Development in Nursing. Philadelphia, F. A. Davis, 1979
20. Newman MA: Editorial. Adv Nurs Sci 5:x–xi, 1983
21. Parse RR: Main-Living-Health: A Theory of Nursing. New York, Wiley, 1981
22. Polit DF, Hungler BF: Nursing Research: Principles and Methods, 2nd ed. Philadelphia, Lippincott, 1983
23. Raile MM: The Relationship of Creativity, Actualization, and Empathy in Unitary Human Development: A Descriptive Study of Rogers's Principle of Helicy, doctoral dissertation, New York University, 1983 (University Microfilms)
24. Rogers ME: An Introduction to the Theoretical Basis of Nursing. Philadelphia, F. A. Davis, 1970
25. Rogers ME: Postulated correlates of unitary human development. New York University, New York, Aug. 22, 1979 (unpublished)
26. Rogers ME: Nursing: A science of unitary man. In Riehl J, Roy C (eds): Conceptual Models for Nursing Practice, 2nd ed. New York, Appleton-Century-Crofts, 1980
27. Rowan J, Reason P: On making sense. In Reason P, Rowan J (eds): Human Inquiry. New York, Wiley, 1981, pp 113–137
28. Shapiro MB: The single case in fundamental clinical psychological research. Br J Med Psychol 34:255–262, 1961
29. Talbot M: Mysticism and the New Physics. New York, Bantam Books, 1980
30. Walizer MH, Wiener PL: Research Methods and Analysis: Searching for Relationships. New York, Harper & Row, Pub, 1976
31. Walker LO, Avant KC: Strategies for Theory Construction in Nursing. Norwalk, Conn, Appleton-Century-Crofts, 1983
32. Wilber K: The problem of proof. ReVision 5:80–100, Spring 1982
33. Wilson LM, Fitzpatrick JJ: Dialectic thinking as a means of understanding systems-in-development: Relevance to Rogers' principles. Adv Nurs Sci 6:24–41, 1984
34. Winstead-Fry P: The scientific method and its impact on holistic health. Adv Nurs Sci 2:1–7, 1980
35. Zukav G: The Dancing Wu Li Masters: An Overview of the New Physics. New York, Morrow, 1979

8

The Relationship Between the Perception of the Speed of Time and the Process of Dying

Marilyn M. Rawnsley

The purpose of this study of the relationship between the perception of the speed of time and the process of dying was to develop testable hypotheses derived from the principles of the holistic theory of nursing proposed by Rogers, in order to address the issue of refutability as one criterion of scientific validity. Four measures of the time experience of 108 subjects, grouped into four categories based on age (younger and older adults) and state (dying or not-dying), were obtained from responses to a time metaphor test, a time-opinion questionnaire, and two verbal estimates of elapsed clock time (20 seconds and 50 seconds). Findings from the study indicate significant differences between groups on certain variables. Younger persons were more oriented to the future and to achievement ($p < 0.05$), while dying persons, who underestimated the 50-second clock interval ($p < 0.05$), also reported more boredom and unhappiness ($p < 0.01$). Other findings suggest a different interpretation of the relationship between the theoretical constructs postulated to describe the human energy field.

BACKGROUND: GENESIS OF PROBLEM FORMULATION

Developing and testing theoretical propositions is a major task of nursing as it advances as a scientific discipline. The theoretical knowledge base of nursing includes both practical and substantive dimensions.[7] Practical or concrete knowledge refers to the use of analogy to make decisions in specific situations based on experience under similar conditions. Substantive knowledge is comprised of abstractions and universals that do not apply to any particular event, but instead provide general principles with wide applicability.[7] It is to the substantive dimension of nursing knowledge that this investigation into the relationship between the perception of the speed of time and the process of dying is addressed.

The purpose of this study was to develop testable hypotheses derived through logical analysis of the assumptions, concepts, and principles of the holistic theory of nursing proposed by Martha E. Rogers.[27] The hypotheses, which examine propositions about increasing complexity and differentiation of the human energy field as it evolves undirectionally along the space–time continuum, were formulated to gain empirical evidence that would verify—or refute—the principle of helicy. Helicy postulates the probabilistic goal-directedness of the life process in humans.[27]

Popper maintained that a theory must be subject to falsification, that is, the concepts must have the potential to be operationalized and empirically tested.[25] Therefore, this study is significant to the substantive domain of nursing knowledge because it speaks to the issue of refutability, which is one criterion for establishing the scientific credibility of a theory.[26]

The study is also significant to the practice dimension of nursing. Choosing to study the time experience of persons who are dying indicates a recognition of the essential connection between nursing research and practice. While nursing is maturing as an academic discipline, it exists historically and functionally as a practice profession committed to promoting the well-being of its patients. Nurses traditionally participate in caring for individuals who are identified as being in a death trajectory.[8] Accurate assessment of the needs of the patient is the premise on which nursing care is planned. Knowledge about the pattern and organization of the human field in the process of dying may change the way in which a dying person's needs are perceived. That is, is it more accurate to describe dying, the final developmental phase of the life process of an individual, as a phenomenon of degradation or entropy, or as a ''period of transition''[27] characterized by increasing differentiation or negentropy? Research designed to examine the time experience of dying persons as a holistic measure of their motion towards entropy or negentropy can yield data that are useful in planning and maintaining a therapeutic milieu for those who are irreversibly moving towards the end of earthly existence. The background literature revealed a philosophical dispute between static and dynamic conceptualizations of space–time.[1, 18, 30] The theoretical positions about the relationships between external or standardized time and psychological or lived time ranged from a hypothetical construct of an internal clock to an explanation of a cognitive-processing-of-information approach.[22, 31]

An inverse relationship between time estimation and metabolic rate has been demonstrated in some studies.[2, 9, 13, 14] Evidence for relationships between time passing and variables such as IQ, socioeconomic status, level of education, and sex of subject has not been consistently demonstrated. A study of body temperature and of personal space failed to correlate body temperature to subjects' production time.[4] Although the notion that time seems to pass faster as people age is generally agreed upon in theoretical writings,[12, 15, 16] empirical findings on the relationship between age and the speed of time passing have been inconclusive.[11, 17, 19, 29] In a study of hospitalized patients, terminally ill subjects underestimated the clock time interval in comparison to suicidal and geriatrically ill subjects.[21]

The problem for study was stated as, "What is the relationship between the perception of the speed of time and the process of dying?" The following assumptions, considered to be logically consistent with Rogerian theory, underlie this study:

1. Chronological age accounts for a difference in the perception of time
2. The dying process is considered to be an irreversible developmental stage of the life process
3. Dying accelerates the rate of exchange of matter and energy between a person and his environment
4. The perception of the speed of time passing reflects the rate of energy exchange between the human field and the environmental field

The hypotheses to be tested in this study were derived from the assumptions of the study and the principles of Rogerian theory, specifically the principle of helicy.[27] They are as follows:

1. Older persons perceive time as passing more swiftly than younger persons
2. Persons who are dying perceive time as passing more swiftly than persons who are not dying
3. Younger persons who are dying perceive time as passing more swiftly than older persons who are not dying
4. There is no relationship between a person's perception of the speed of time passing and his or her estimation of an interval of clock time

The theoretical and operational definitions of the terms of this study were:

Theoretical	**Operational**
Dying:	
A state or condition that is presumed irreversible and precedes the cessation of life	Persons who have a confirmed diagnosis of metastatic cancer
Not-Dying:	
Any state or condition of the human field that does not threaten its survival	Persons who are not diagnosed as having a life-threatening illness
Older Persons:	
Individuals who are presumed to be in the developmental life stage of later adulthood	Persons who are between the ages of 55 and 75[12]

82 THEORY AND RESEARCH

Theoretical	Operational
Younger Persons:	
Individuals who are presumed to be in the developmental life stage of early adulthood	Persons who are between the ages of 17 and 30[12, 24]
Perception of the Speed of Time Passing:	
The individual's personal experience of change	The score obtained on the Time Metaphor Test and/or on the Speed of Time Passing variable of the Time Opinion Survey[16, 17]
Underestimation of Clock Time:	
The judgment of an interval of clock time as less than (shorter than) the actual amount of time that has elapsed according to the clock[6]	A verbal response of less than 20 seconds on the first elapsed interval and/or a response of less than 50 seconds on the second elapsed interval
Overestimation of Clock Time:	
The judgment of an interval of clock time as greater than (longer than) the actual amount of time that has elapsed according to the clock[6, 15]	A verbal response of more than 20 seconds on the first elapsed interval and/or a verbal response of more than 50 seconds on the 50-second elapsed interval

RELATIONSHIP TO THE SCIENCE OF UNITARY HUMAN BEINGS

From the assumptions, concepts, and principles of the holistic theory of nursing proposed by Rogers,[27] certain relationships between the variables of age, state of human energy field, and perception of the speed of time were predicted. Rogers postulates a complementarity of *"man"* and *environment* in which the fundamental unit of life is an energy field. Accordingly, *"man,"* an open system, is conceptualized as a human energy field possessing a characteristic pattern and organization. This human energy field is continuously simultaneously interacting with the environmental energy field, both of which are embedded in a four-dimensional matrix composed of the three dimensions of space and the further dimension of time. Such mutual simultaneous interaction involves exchange of matter and energy across the contiguous, fluctuating boundaries of these fields. Furthermore, Rogers holds that the life process in *"man"* evolves unidirectionally and irreversibly along the space–time continuum in the direction of increasing complexity or differentiation of the pattern and organization of the field. As the human field expands into the environmental field, there is presumed to be an increase in the size of the human field and a decrease in its density accompanied by a blurring of boundaries between fields. All of these changes occur as the human field ages and are associated with a perception of time as seeming to pass more quickly.[27]

Therefore, if the life process is unidirectional and irreversible in the direction of increasing differentiation and complexity, and if this evolutionary process of aging is associated with a perception of time passing quickly, then older persons would have a faster time perception than younger persons (hypothesis 1). A further interpretation of the theory led to the assumption that the dying process was characterized by an acceleration of the changes associated with aging. It was reasoned that if the life process were irreversible, and dying were a developmental phase of that life process, then in dying, the changes in size and density of the human field would be accelerated as the human boundary became less distinct from the environmental boundary. Consequently, it was presumed that persons who were dying would perceive time as passing more swiftly than persons who were not dying (hypothesis 2). Finally, it was reasoned that if the dying process accelerated the changes in the human field beyond the rate experienced in aging, then young persons who were dying would report a faster time perception than older persons who were not dying (hypothesis 3).

Time is a phenomenon experienced by the whole individual. That is, regardless of whether a particular stimulus or incident can be categorized as biological, intellectual, or emotional, it is translated into the time experience of the person as a whole.[23] Thus, time experience as felt by the individual is a holistic phenomenon and as such can be considered an appropriate measure for testing Rogers' holistic theory.

The perception of time passing (PTP) is directly related to exchange between the two fields and may be stated in symbolic form as:

$$\text{PTP} = f\,\text{MSI}\left(\text{M}\left\|\left\|\frac{m + e}{\underset{\longleftarrow}{\overset{\longrightarrow}{m + e}}}\right\|\right\|\text{E}\right)$$

According to this symbolic representation, perception of time passing is a function of the mutual simultaneous interaction (MSI) of the human field (M) and environmental field (E) involving an exchange ($\rightleftarrows$) of matter and energy ($m + e$) across fluctuating boundaries ($\|$). Therefore, the rate of exchange of matter and energy between fields is reflected in the speed with which time is perceived to be passing. Dying has been assumed to be an acceleration of the rate of exchange between fields across boundaries that are becoming increasingly blurred. The relationship of the perception of time passing and dying is symbolically stated thus:

$$\text{D} = dc\,(\text{LP}) \rightarrow \uparrow\,(r) \qquad \left(\text{M}\underset{m + e}{\overset{m + e}{\rightleftarrows}}\text{E}\right) \rightarrow \frac{\text{PTP}}{sw}$$

This symbolic representation states that dying (D) is a developmental correlate (dc) of the life process (LP) characterized by an acceleration of the rate ($\uparrow r$) of exchange of matter and energy ($m + e$) across blurring boundaries ($\|$) between the human field (M) and the environmental field (E), leading to a perception of time passing swiftly. Therefore, the question for study that examined the relationship between the perception of the speed of time and the process of dying represents a logical deduction from the theory. If persons who were dying perceived time as passing more swiftly than persons who were not dying, then it could be inferred that there was an acceleration of the rate of exchange of matter and energy between fields.

Two dimensions of time experience are the perception of felt or experiential time and the assessment of a standardized objective measure of clock time.[5] Felt or experiential time has been referred to in the literature as the inner time sense of the individual as he or she experiences change, as psychological time, and as lived time.[3, 10, 20] Felt time is defined as progressive or unidirectional change toward continuing advance such as growth. Cyclic time can be measured by an objective means such as estimation or production of an interval of clock time, while progressive time is assessed from the responses of the individual who is experiencing it.[28] In this study perception of time passing referred to the progressive time experience, which is synonymous with felt or experiential time. It was predicted that data about progressive time experience would not be correlated with data about clock time experience (hypothesis 4).

METHOD

The sample was comprised of 108 subjects, 41 men and 67 women, who could read and write English. Subjects were selected from inpatient settings so that the environments, although not controlled according to laboratory standards, were similar. Subjects were categorized on the basis of age and state into four groups:

> Group A—Older, Dying—30 persons between the ages of 55 and 75 with a diagnosis of metastatic cancer
> Group B—Older, Not-Dying—30 persons between the ages of 55 and 75 with a non-life-threatening diagnosis
> Group C—Younger, Dying—18 persons between the ages of 17 and 30 with a diagnosis of metastatic cancer
> Group D—Younger, Not-Dying—30 persons between the ages of 17 and 30 with a non-life-threatening diagnosis

All of the subjects in Group C and 24 subjects in Group A were aware of the diagnosis of cancer. Awarenes of diagnosis was determined in two ways: first, nursing staff were asked whether or not the patient had been told of the diagnosis; secondly, after the testing session was completed, the patient was asked what brought him or her to the hospital.

Two instruments were used to measure subjects' perceptions about time. The first tool consists of 25 metaphors or phrases that a poet might use to symbolize time. Knapp and Garbutt developed this *Time Metaphor Test* in order to study relationships between time imagery and the achievement motive.[16] Two separate factor analyses of these metaphors have yielded one factor, *swift to static* meaning of time.[17, 21]

Subjects were instructed to choose the five metaphors from the list that most closely stated how time seemed to be passing in their lives. Using the weight assigned to each item by Wallach and Green, each subject's total score was computed by adding the rank number of the item. The higher the total score, the faster the perception of time.[29] The procedure of having subjects select the five metaphors most appropriate to them represents a different methodology from that previously reported in the literature. This method has the advantage of being simpler for ill and elderly subjects to complete than previous methods of ranking all 25 items, yet it reflects the subject's preference for swift or static metaphors.

The second instrument, *The Time Opinion Survey,* was devised by Kuhlen and Monge to be a more direct method of assessment of time experience than the metaphor test.[17] This tool, which consists of multiple-choice items constructed to form an approximate interval scale, yields five factors said to be linked to perceived rate of time passing: the speed of time passage (STP); future orientation and achievement (FOA); feelings of time pressure (TP); ability to delay gratification (DG); and current life conditions (CLC).[17] The third measure of time experience was the behavioral method of estimation of two elapsed intervals of clock time, 20 seconds and 50 seconds. There is controversy in the literature about the meaning of different methods of clock time estimation.[6, 22] Doob's rationale that verbal estimation assesses the lived or felt time experience of the individual was accepted. He clarified research methods in current use: a verbal underestimation means that time feels as if it were passing quickly; a verbal overestimation means that time feels as if it were passing slowly.[6]

The tests were administered in individual sessions by one of six research assistants—who were unaware of the hypotheses—in the following order: the Time Metaphor Test; the Time Opinion Survey; verbal estimation of two elapsed intervals, 20 seconds, then 50 seconds. All research protocols of the five participating hospitals were followed, and subjects gave written consent to participate.

Because of the purposive sampling method, the findings of the study cannot be generalized beyond the sample. However, there is no reason to conclude that this sample differs in any important ways from other persons hospitalized for similar conditions.

RESULTS

To determine the predictions of the first three hypotheses, data were analyzed by a one-way analysis of variance. The results did not support the first hypothesis; however, a trend in the opposite direction was noted. The second hypothesis was partially supported; subjects who were dying underestimated the 50-second elapsed interval ($p, <0.05$). The third hypothesis was not supported. Instead, findings revealed Group B (older, not-dying) and Group C (younger, dying) to be more alike in their perception of the speed of time passing than any other combination of groups (B, $\overline{X} = 4.66$; C, $\overline{X} = 4.63$).

Data on the fourth hypothesis were analyzed by the Pearson Product Moment Correlation. Findings obtained from correlation of the Time Metaphor Test Scores with the 20-second elapsed interval (R = 0.01) and the 50-second elapsed interval (R = 0.05) were not significant; there was no relationship demonstrated between a subject's perception of the speed of time passing (felt time) and the estimation of an interval of clock time (cyclic time).

Other significant findings were that future orientation and achievement are developmental concepts related to age of subjects, as younger persons (Groups C and D), regardless of diagnosis, were more future-oriented ($p < 0.05$); and that dying persons (Groups A and C) reported more unhappiness and boredom in life ($p < 0.01$).

The predictions of the first three hypotheses were deduced from the theoretical propositions about increasing complexity and differentiation being accompanied by change in the size and density of the human field as it expands into the environmental field. Time seeming to pass quickly was associated with these shifts in the human field patterns[27] as matter and energy were postulated to be more rapidly exchanged across field boundaries that were becoming increasingly blurred.

That interpretation of increasing complexity must take into account the findings of this study, which suggest different relationships among the field variables of age, state, size, density, and boundary. Table 8–1 illustrates these relationships.

DISCUSSION

In light of the findings, it seems that there are two interrelated constructs essential to increasing complexity: expansion of the human field into the environmental field and motion of the field. It is further suggested that the expanded size of the field, with the concomitant decrease in density and blurring of boundaries, is accompanied by a shift in the pattern of energy exchange between persons and environment. That is, as the human field increases in complexity through the gradual process of aging, the field boundary may change from rather nonspecific incorporation of matter and energy in the young, less differentiated field to an actively selective process in the older, more differentiated field. Likewise, younger persons who are dying are increasing in complexity at an accelerated rate in comparison with their chronological peers. Therefore, their field boundaries are more similar to the actively selective field boundaries of the older, nondying adults. Finally, well-differentiated fields of older, dying adults perceive time as passing slowly, since their field boundaries, which are highly discriminating in regard to the less differentiated environment, are integrating only those energy patterns that are complementary.

One assumption of this study was that perception of time passing reflects the rate of energy exchange between fields. Thus, it was postulated that changes in field boundaries are accompanied by a shift in the pattern of energy input and output.

TABLE 8–1. RELATIONSHIPS AMONG FIELD VARIABLES

Field Characteristics	Group A	Group B	Group C	Group D
Age and state	55–75 ($\overline{X} = 64.1$ years) Dying	55–75 ($\overline{X} = 64.7$ years) Not-Dying	17–30 ($\overline{X} = 21$ years) Dying	17–30 ($\overline{X} = 24$ years) Not-Dying
Size and density	Almost fully expanded into environment; highly diffuse, complex patterning under conditions of aging and dying	Moderately expanded and diffuse; increasing complexity of patterning relative to aging process	Moderately expanded and diffuse; increasing complexity of patterning relative to dying process	Less expanded and more dense and less complexity of patterning relative to Groups A, B, C
Boundary of field	Blurred, highly discriminating	Blurring, actively selective	Blurring, actively selective	More distinct; nonselective
Process or motion of expansion	Slow, nearly complete	Expanding, gradually and cumulatively re aging	Expanding; accelerated re dying	Dynamically involved in motion of expansion
Pattern of energy exchange between fields	Integrates only complementary patterning slow rate of exchange	Incorporates a wider variety of energy patterns than A; less than D; moderate rate	Incorporates a wider variety of patterns than A; less than D; moderate rate	Nondiscriminating incorporation of energy exchange—rapid rate
Predicted time perception	Swiftest	Swifter than D; not as swift as A and C	Swifter than B and D; not as swift as A	Slowest
Reported time perception (STP)	Slowest ($\overline{X} = 4$)	Almost the same as Group C; slower than D; faster than A ($\overline{X} = 4.63$)	Almost the same as Group B; slower than D; faster than A ($\overline{X} = 4.66$)	Swiftest ($\overline{X} = 5.23$)
Reported 50-second clock interval	Slightly overestimated ($\overline{X} = 53.5$)	Greatly overestimated ($\overline{X} = 84.0$)	Slightly overestimated ($\overline{X} = 57.8$)	Greatly overestimated ($\overline{X} = 80.6$)

Postulating a shift in the pattern of energy exchange between fields explains the finding that dying persons, regardless of age, underestimated the elapsed clock interval. Instructions were given to each subject before the clock exercise began that they were not to count to themselves, tap their fingers, or talk. Radios or televisions were turned off, and only the subject and the research assistant were in the room. In effect, available input from the environmental field was diminished. Therefore, verbal estimation of the elapsed clock interval may have been an expression of energy output when input was reduced. That is, the dying field continued to release energy regardless of environmental input as it inevitably moved toward completion of the life process.

Rethinking the conceptual relationships between the constructs of size, density, boundary, and motion of the human field lends a different perspective to the problem of what it is like to be dying. If the dying field is highly differentiated and discriminating in regard to environmental energy patterns, how can therapeutic milieu be fostered for persons moving toward the end of the life process? Is the hospice concept more appropriate for a highly differentiated, highly discriminating dying field than hospital settings that prioritize technology, efficiency, and procedure above individualized patient care? How might the construct of patterning shifts in energy exchange between fields relate to the type of population being served, to environmental overload or deprivation, and to staff burnout?

From the new world view postulated by the Rogerian science, there are countless questions to be asked, problems to be studied, measurements to be devised, and scholarly positions to be argued. What this study of the relationship of the speed of time and the process of dying has demonstrated is that testable hypotheses can be devised from Rogerian theory and examined empirically. Thus, by addressing and meeting the criterion of refutability, a new direction for the scientific study of Roger's holistic theory of nursing has begun.

REFERENCES

1. Brillocin L: The arrow of time. In Zeman J (ed): Time in Science and Philosophy. New York, Elsevier, 1971
2. Cohen J: Psychological Time in Health and Disease. Springfield, Ill, Charles C Thomas, 1967
3. Cohen J: Time is psychology. In Zeman J (ed): Time in Science and Philosophy. New York, Elsevier, 1971
4. Collett B: Variations in body temperature, perceived duration and perceived personal space. Int J Nurs Stud 11:47–60, 1971
5. Cottle T: The location of experience: A manifest time orientation. Acta Psychol (Amst) 2:129–149, 1968
6. Doob L: Patterning of Time. New Haven, Yale University Press, 1971
7. Duffy M, Muhlenkamp A: A framework for theory analysis. Nurs Outlook 22:570–574, 1974
8. Epstein C: Nursing the Dying Patient. Reston,Va, Prentice-Hall, 1975

9. Fischer R: Biological time. In Fraser JT (ed): The Voices of Time. New York, George Braziller, 1966, pp 357–382

10. Fraisse P: The Psychology of Time. New York, Harper & Row, Pub, 1963

11. Fink H: The relationship of time perspective to age, institutionalization and activity. J Gerontol 12:414–417, 1957

12. Gould R: The phases of adult life: A study in developmental psychology. Am J Psychiatry 72:521–531, 1972

13. Hoagland H: The physiological control of judgements of duration: Evidence for a chemical clock. J Genetic Psychology 9:267–287, 1933

14. Hoagland H: Some biochemical considerations of time. In Fraser JT (ed): The Voices of Time. New York, George Braziller, 1966, pp 312–329

15. Holubar J: The Sense of Time. Cambridge, Mass, MIT Press, 1969

16. Knapp R, Garbutt J: Time imagery and the achievement motive. J Pers 26:426–434, 1959

17. Kuhlen R, Monge R: Correlates of estimated rate of time passage in the adult years. J Gerontol 23:427–433, 1968

18. LeShan L: Human survival of biological death. Main Currents Mod Thought 25:35–45, 1969

19. Lynch D: Future time perspective and impulsivity in old age. J Genet Psychol 118:245–252, 1971

20. Minkowski E: Lived Time. Evanston, Ill, Northwestern University Press, 1970

21. Neuringer C, Harris R: The perception of the passage of time in death-involved hospital patients. Life Threat Behav 1:240–254, 1974

22. Newman N: Time estimation in relation to gait tempo. Percept Mot Skills 34:359–366, 1972

23. Ornstein R: On the Experience of Time. Baltimore, Penguin Books, 1969

24. Piaget J: Time perception in children. In Fraser JT (ed): The Voices of Time. New York, George Braziller, 1966, pp 202–216

25. Popper K: The Logic of Scientific Discovery. New York, Harper Torchbook, 1968

26. Quine WV, Ullian JS: The Web of Belief. New York, Random House, 1970

27. Rogers ME: Introduction to the Theoretical Basis of Nursing. Philadelphia, FA Davis, 1971

28. Schlegal R: Time and entropy. In Zeman J (ed): Time in Science and Philosophy. New York, Elsevier, 1971

29. Wallach M, Green L: On age and the subjective speed of time. J Gerontol 16:71–74, 1961

30. Watanabe S: Creative time. In Fraser J, Haber H, Muller G (eds): The Study of Time. New York, Springer-Verlag, 1972, pp 159–188

31. Zelkind I: Factors in time estimation and a case for the internal clock. J Genet Psychol 88: 295–301, 1973

Critique of Rawnsley's Study

Joyce J. Fitzpatrick

Rogers' postulations regarding the developmental process have provided consistent intrigue for the Rogerian student. Specifically, investigators have concerned themselves with phylogenetic and ontogenetic processes characterized by increased complexity and diversity. A more specific postulate of Rogers' was that perception of time was a developmental correlate. Thus, as persons proceeded in development, they moved from a perception of time passing slowing through time passing rapidly to a sense of timelessness.

With this general background, Rawnsley studied the relationship between perception of time and the process of dying. But she went further, to include also those who were not-dying, both young and old, just as she included young and old dying persons. Thus, the study has incorporated in it an evaluation of the ontogenetic developmental process, specifically in relation to speed of time passage. Because of the need to conform to the research process, Rawnsley simplified her problem statement, and thus understated the conceptual complexity of her work.

The logical connections between Rogers' assumptions and postulates regarding human development and time and Rawnsley's derivations of relationships, as reflected in the hypotheses, appeared to be a major contribution of this work. What should be added here is a clear explication of the theoretical links between Rogers' assumptions and the relationships posited by Rawnsley.

Rawnsley proposed that the hypotheses were derived through the logical analysis of the assumptions, concepts, and principles explicated by Rogers. (To include all of this in one study would be a major scientific accomplishment, and a major study.) A major problem in this study was the detailed specification of the logical analysis that occurred. Rawnsley's arguments were more general and lacked strong theoretical or empirical support. For example, in justifying the use of the concept "time," Rawnsley proposed that it "is a phenomenon experienced by the whole individual." Not only was this major tenet unsupported, but also the use of time terms was inconsistent. It was not always clear that the investigator was concerned about the perception of time. She varied in selection of labels to describe the time concept. This lack of precision in terminology was also reflected in the instruments selected and the measurements used. (One was not always certain that the investigator had clearly specified the concepts, the variables, and the operational definitions.) Rather, Rawnsley described the theoretical links in general terms. The presentation of the relationship to the Science of Unitary Human Beings could have been strengthened by the provision of supporting documentation or by a more thorough explication of the steps of the logical analysis that occurred.

Rawnsley could more strongly justify the selection of her measurements of time. There appeared in fact to be a great deal of ambiguity in the cited literature regarding various definitions of time.

Rawnsley did not clearly link her instruments to the variables. It was difficult to thoroughly evaluate the methodological aspects of this research because of the brevity of the report. However, it appears that the study could be considerably strengthened by a refinement in methodology and study design.

Rawnsley provided an interesting idea about the links to professional practice. This dimension could be further elaborated. In a period of high concern for innovative nursing interventions, this translation into practice could be most enlightening to those nurses searching for alternative modalities for enhancing health.

Critique of Rawnsley's Study

Helen M. Ference

Rawnsley's study of 1977 was the initial test of Rogers' Science of Unitary Human Beings. While other studies had addressed the issue of time, this is the first known work to use Rogers' framework in its totality, as Rogers had described it in 1970. Given this extreme limitation, Rawnsley set out to define operationally the speed of time and the process of dying, according to a four-dimensional framework. Her findings provided a basis for dialogue among serious researchers who sought to verify the principles of human synergistic development proposed by Rogers.

In this study, the hypothesis that older persons perceive time passing more swiftly than younger persons was not supported. Rather, a trend in the opposite direction was found. This finding raised the question of the meaning of chronological age or linear time, as it is perceived in a four-dimensional framework. Human development, in a three-dimensional framework, is defined according to linear time. In this perspective chronological age has meaning. In contrast, a four-dimensional framework assumes that time is relative in the space–time continuum; hence, time is unrelated to clock time. Logically, therefore, it seems that energy field evolvement in a space–time continuum is identifiable by more and/or different variables than chronological age. These results encourage investigators to redefine the evolution of unitary human beings according to the complexity and diversity of the field pattern, rather than by chronological age. This exploration may help us to understand why some people appear "older" than others of the same chronological age.

It appears that Rawnsley's categories of "dying" and "not-dying" may not be mutually exclusive. The operational definitions of dying (diagnosis of metastatic cancer) and not-dying (no life-threatening illness) may be exclusive according to medical definition. However, dying is a transition process of the energy field, according to Rogers. Therefore, in the Rogerian framework other field manifestations of this transition process may be functioning. For instance, the young, not-dying group of patients was hospitalized during a transitional stage of their lives. Late teenage and early adulthood energy fields may be high frequency, where the pattern is transforming to a more evolved level of diversity. The four study groups may have been too homogeneous to demonstrate mean differences on the instruments measuring the perception of time passing. Rawnsley does suggest a trend that the dying groups perceived time as passing more quickly than the nondying groups, regardless of chronological age. Perhaps a broader definition of transition should be considered before operationally defining one manifestation of that process, which is dying.

As in any beginning study, definitions bring specificity to the new language and constructs. Redefinitions begin to unfold. This has been the case in the Science of Unitary Human Beings. Since Rogers' first edition of *The Theoretical Framework of Nursing* (1970), upon which Rawnsley's study is based, several terms have been modified. ''Unidirectionality'' has been determined to be inconsistent with multidimensionality. Even though the direction of evolution has not been changed, the term is no longer used, as it did not contribute to the understanding of the conceptual system. Rawnsley's study results helped with this redefinition. Also, the term ''boundaries'' is no longer used within the framework. Boundaries of an energy field tend to confuse the basic assumption of openness. In Rogers' framework, the energy field is not relatively open or closed; it is completely open. Further, the term *mutual simultaneous interaction,* as referred to by Rawnsley, was later changed to *continuous mutual process.* The former term suggested a temporal orientaion of human and environmental energy fields, rather than a four-dimensional, space–time perspective.

In summary, Rawnsley's work, completed at Boston University, is considered to be the research that initiated empirical testing of Rogers' framework. Two major issues addressed here were based upon her findings. The first issue is the utility of chronological age as an index of unitary human beings. The second issue is the theoretical definition of energy field transition that will support the operational definition of dying. Rawnsley's study provided a scientific legitimacy to further empirical investigation of the Science of Unitary Human Beings.

Response
Marilyn M. Rawnsley

In reading the separate critiques of my study on time and dying, I am struck by the obvious difference in the focus of each reviewer. Fitzpatrick's critique challenges the methods of the study primarily in regard to the derivation of the hypotheses and the links established between the measurements of time and the constructs of the Rogerian conceptual system. In contrast, Ference addresses the substantive issues that were raised in response to the findings of the study.

While I can understand her concern with methodological rigor, I find Fitzpatrick's analysis rather elaborate for a study whose value lies in its historical relevance—rather than in its contemporary meaning—to the Science of Unitary Human Beings. The brevity of a research report mitigates against "the more thorough explication of the steps of the logical analysis" Fitzpatrick requests. However, serious students of Rogers' conceptual system are referred to the dissertation from which this study is excerpted in order to examine its logical adequacy. Discussion of the methodological problems may be more appropriate as an academic exercise in doctoral seminars. For, in light of the changes in the Rogerian conceptual system in the several years since this study was completed, the question is, as they say, moot.

In response to the critique written by Ference, I can express only my appreciation for her objectivity. Since her own research clarified some of the problems apparent in my study, I am particularly interested in her insights and interpretations about the theoretical meaning of my work. In analyzing the study within its historical context, she acknowledges its inherent limitations without dismissing its heuristic value to the emerging Science of Unitary Human Beings.

Ference suggests that this study "provided a basis for dialogue among serious researchers" committed to the Rogerian framework. Scientific knowledge advances through the perpetuation of inquiry; scientists question, refine, and redefine the problems studied by their predecessors. If the curiosity and the controversy aroused by my study spurred further inquiry into the Science of Unitary Human Beings, I am honored.

9

The Relationship of Time Experience, Creativity Traits, Differentiation, and Human Field Motion

Helen M. Ference

The principle of resonancy has been verified by the findings reported in this study. Four indices are confirmed as measures of human synergistic development. Human field motion was found to be related to three other indices of human synergistic development: creativity, differentiation, and time experience. The human field motion tool was supported as a valid measure, as well as the first instrument developed for the purpose of assessing four-dimensional, whole man according to the Science of Unitary Man.

BACKGROUND: GENESIS OF PROBLEM FORMULATION

It is seemingly odd and sometimes difficult to refer to the person, generically called "man," as a human energy field. Many of us have been taught to think that an energy field is a paranormal phenomenon or a freak, nonhuman thing. It is difficult to look at ourselves in a different way. The different view may be in conflict with our values, beliefs, and feelings. But should such a conflict be a reason to deny this way of knowing ourselves and furthering our understanding of mankind? This study is based upon the Science of Unitary Man,[26, 27] where generic man is a human energy field. This science provides a new way of understanding human behavior.

Certainly, many university courses have presented material that challenge our views of the world. Few students of nursing have never come in conflict with a health notion studied in their nursing programs. Myths are altered; parent teachings are challenged. It seems that the world of education belittles the rules that formulated our development and guided us through life events. But such is the nature of science.

New research findings can be startling. They challenge us to look at our old ways of functioning, to decide their merit, and to move on to new frontiers. A new focus can provide us with an understanding of behaviors that have previously been unexplained. Accepting a new focus is necessary for our comprehension of four-dimensional man and human synergistic development.

Motion has been associated with growth and development for many years. Rocking is known to increase physiological development of infants.[11, 20, 25] Rocking also increases the social performance of the elderly. Imposed motion, in the form of transportation, either enhances our outlook on life or tires us out. Jogging, as a form of motion, either slows people down or speeds them up. Some people prefer to jog in the morning, while others feel better when they jog in the afternoon. This feeling is most likely due to their human field motion position.

Motion is valued as positive when it enhances our well-being, that is, when we feel good in relation to the motion. When we experience disharmony in the motion, the motion is valued as negative. Motion can be compared to the activity–rest concept, which is a dichotomous way of looking at the motion of three-dimensional man. Human field motion is an ever-present phenomenon of the four-dimensional human energy field. In its low frequency position it resembles rest. In its higher frequency position is resembles activity. Rest and activity may not be related to physical motion. Another aspect of apparent motion is related to the environmental energy field. For example, a child in a high frequency position may appear hyperactive when functioning in a low frequency environment. On the other hand, the same child may not appear to be hyperactive in a multistimuli, high frequency environment.

RELATIONSHIP TO THE SCIENCE OF UNITARY HUMAN BEINGS

This study is an empirical investigation of Rogers' construct of human synergistic development. What is human synergistic development, and how does it differ from human development as we commonly think of it? Human synergistic development (HSD) is a "dynamic, multidimensional, unique behavior of whole systems and a negentropic process characterized by increasing complexity and diversity of energy field pattern and organization."[26, 27] In contrast, human development is commonly referred to as the growth and maturation of the physical and psychological being. There is a physical acceleration until adulthood, followed by a gradual wearing down of the physiological systems until death. The basic difference between the two constructs stems from our view of the world. Human synergistic development is based in a four-dimensional view of the world where space–time is relative. Human development, as we commonly think of it, is based in a three-dimensional view of the world, where height, depth, and width are physical coordinates that define the boundaries of man.

Synergistic development represents the whole, being different from the sum of its parts. The outcomes of synergistic development are holistic, new, and innovatively different. In contrast, the development of outcomes in a three-dimensional focus are homeostatic and reflect a previous state of equilibrium. The two approaches differ. The synergistic, four-dimensional view demands use of the process of synthesis, whereas the three-dimensional, nonsynergistic focus demands that we use analysis and reduce man to the study of his parts, such as his physiology or psychology. The human is unable to maintain both perceptions of reality simultaneously. For purposes of developing the Science of Unitary Man and its specific language, the four-dimensional approach has been accepted. Comprehending research that is derived from Rogers' Science of Unitary Man[28] requires a basic understanding of four-dimensionality and space–time relativity.

This study was designed to verify the principle of resonancy, according to the framework of the Science of Unitary Man. It was hypothesized that there is a relationship between human field motion and human synergistic development according to the principle of resonancy. For many years (1970–77), Rogers had reported observations in support of the notion that the human field develops in the direction of low frequency, long energy wave forms to high frequency, short energy wave forms. Rogers referred to these observations as "correlates of synergistic human development." The principle of resonancy is based on these observations and states that generic man evolves in the direction of higher frequency and shorter energy waves. Rogers' observations were unrefined and could not serve as operational definitions of human synergistic development.

This study was the first attempt to specify these observations as "the correlates of development" and as mutually exclusive indices of the human energy field, as well as to determine their relationship to each other. For the first time, there was an actual, empirical measure of the human energy field. This was a measure of human field motion. The Human Field Motion Tool provided researchers with a new way of studying man. The measure of human field motion is an index of whole man, where the whole is different from the sum of the parts.

Theoretical Evolution of Human Field Motion

As the investigator searched the literature for studies and discussion of motion, it was apparent that motion has been investigated from three-dimensional perspectives. Because the Science of Unitary Man is based in a four-dimensional framework and is the framework for this study, contrasting views of motion according to three-dimensionality and four-dimensionality are discussed for a clearer understanding.

Three-dimensional motion studies have focused on the human functions of eye movements,[2] visual perception of rotary motion,[4] and color and brightness.[12] Although notable contributions in the physical and psychological sciences, the findings cannot be used to explain the development of unitary man.

Four-dimensionality assumes that space–time is a synthesis of space and time coordinates.[5, 39] This contrasts with the three-dimensionl approach of reducing the components of space and time for analysis. There is support for investigating motion in four-dimensionality. For example, Kolers[16] suggested that the existing motion theories were inadequate because time's role has not been clarified. Also, Bondy[3] speculated that visual shape and motion in different events are meaningfully different because some individuals perceive more than the singular shape or motion, such as the combination of both. Her suggestion that perception varies in different environments supports a mutual process of human and environment energy fields. These postulations served as a basis for investigating motion in a four-dimensional perspective.

Rogers[27] postulated that the human energy field wave frequency is higher with increasing motion. In order to specify motion for empirical study in the Science of Unitary Man,[26, 28] the author designated this index "human field motion" and theoretically defined it as an experiential, multidimensional position.[13]

Capra has stated that "the particle's state of motion is contained in the wave length and frequency of that wave. . . ."[5] Comparing this statement to the level of unitary "man," we find a similar meaning of motion determined by the principle of resonancy.[26, 28] A description of human field motion according to wave frequency requires a different set of reference points from spatial and clock-time objects. An expression of human field motion arises from man's feelings. Reports of " . . . merging action and awareness,"[10] flow experience,[10] and "peak experiences"[18] are characteristic of this feeling. There is an intense absorption of oneself with little regard for clock-time or three-dimensional objects. With high frequency human field motion it is not uncommon to seem "unresponsive" to physical environmental events, such as people entering the room or phones ringing. There is a sense of exuberance, sometimes followed by a relaxing and revitalized feeling. The author speculates that high frequency human field motion contributes to the complexity and diversity of the human field pattern.

The term *human field motion* originates from Rogers'[27] postulated field manifestations of field expansion, lightness, and less visibility. Colloquialisms used to describe this experience are "My motor is running," "What a drag," "I'm flying or really moving." Operational definitions of feelings can employ symbolic drawings,[30] or word expression of meaning. The semantic differential technique[23, 24] is a word expression technique that was selected for the tool development of human field motion.

The Human Field Motion Tool was developed and pilot tested in 1978. The tool that was pilot tested consisted of 23 scales reported by Osgood and Suci[23, 24] and nine additional bipolar words found to be associated with lower and higher wave frequency according to Rogers' conceptual system of synergistic human development. Five judges confirmed the face validity and relative direction of the bipolar descriptors. In the pilot study, 43 subjects rated 3 concepts against 32 scales. Retest reliability was performed on 4 percent of the items, and internal consistency was determined for the scales by concepts. The scales having lowest correlation with one another across concepts were selected to minimize interactional effects. Two concepts and 13 scales were retained as a measure of human field motion. Since some scales were rated on both concepts, the total number of independent scales in the tool are 20.

The Human Field Motion Tool was submitted to 213 subjects in the main study and factor analyzed. Three factors typically emerge when the semantic differential technique is used. Three factors emerged as predicted, and each scale loaded on at least one factor. All scales are in the same direction of wave frequency as specified by the judges. This analysis provides factorial validity of the tool and supports the principle of resonancy. Retest reliability is 0.77 in the pilot test and 0.70 in the main study. The part-whole correlations of each scale ranged from 0.51 to 0.77. The correlation of the score of each concept to the total test score is 0.87 for both concepts of "my motor is running" and "my field expansion."

Human Synergistic Development

In this study, human synergistic development was defined as the interrelated set of time experience, differentiation, and creativity traits. These indices were specified from Rogers' proposed correlates that development is in the direction of (1) time racing, (2) more differentiation, and (3) more imagination.

Time experience is the perception of time passing as measured by the Knapp and Garbutt[15] Time Metaphor Test. The swift-to-static factor described by Wallach and Green[34] was assumed to support factorial validity. The K-R 20 measure of reliabiity is 0.99 in this study.

Creativity traits are attributes of the creative person as measured by a 19-adjective scale by Domino[8] from the Adjective Check List.[14] The K-R 20 measure of reliability in this study is 0.98. A comparison of adjectives from the Adjective Check List was made with a 27-item scale[31] and an 8-item scale[31] and those that correlate with the Barron-Welsh Art Scale.[1] Through this comparative analysis, the 19-item scale was determined to be the most reflective of the creative person.

Differentiation is increasing complexity and diversity and heterogeneity[13] as measured by Witkin's[36] Group Embedded Figures Test. Rogers[26] defines "negentropy" as "increasing heterogeneity, differentiation, diversity, complexity of pattern and organization." Rogers also postulates that development is negentropic and that the direction of that development is toward greater differentiation. The use of *differentiation* by Witkin and Rogers is quite similar, and thereby this term was accepted by the investigator as a valid theoretical and operational definition. Alternate forms reliability in this study for the Group Embedded Figures Test is 0.79.

Hypothesis

It was hypothesized that there is a relationship between human synergistic development and human field motion. Set theory was used to ascertain the relationship between two sets of variables. These variables are the operational definitions of the theoretical indices of human synergistic development.

The first set was creativity, differentiation, and time experience, which was referred to as "the human synergistic development (HSD) set." The second set was 20 scales of human field motion, referred to as "the human field motion (HFM) set."

The HSD set had construct validity, since each variable was being measured by well-established tools. The HFM scales, on the other hand, had face validity and factorial validity. The purpose of relating the two sets was to substantiate human field motion as a necessary variable in the definition of human synergistic development.

METHOD

A canonical correlation design was employed to ascertain the canonical relations between the two composite sets of variables. The independent variable set is human synergistic development, and the dependent variable set is human field motion.

The population is men and women between the chronological ages of 30 and 60 years who read and write in the English language. The age delimitation was selected because two tests have been known to show differences when administered to subjects who are outside of this age range. There are known differences by sex below the age of 30 on the Group Embedded Figures Test, and there are reported scale-checking differences on the semantic differential technique beyond the chronological age of 60.

The sample size is 213, which is sufficient to detect a medium effect size in the population with a power of 0.75 at the 0.05 level of significance.[6] The sampling frame is national conferences or meetings.

Data collection was done in groups with specified directions for the data collectors. It took subjects approximately 45 minutes to 1 hour to complete a consent form, a demographic information sheet, and four paper-pencil tests.

RESULTS

The hypothesis is supported. Three canonical variates emerge: the first, named complexity-diversity pattern, has a canonical R of 0.41 at a 0.001 level of significance; the second, named human field motion, has a canonical R of 0.37 at a 0.01 level of significance; and a third that is not named because it is not significant at the 0.05 level, has a canonical R of 0.33 at a 0.07 level of significance. The contention that when three dimensions are held constant, the two sets are independent is not supported, since only 42 percent of the variance is accounted for by those three dimensions. This result suggests that either the variable sets are insufficient or the instruments are insufficient to measure the variables. Forty-two percent of the variance is, however, a large percentage considering the nature of the research.

It was hypothesized that the correlated sets of indices of human synergistic development are complete. Applying a mathematical model meant that the variance would be fully accounted for by the two sets of variables. This is a lofty hypothesis. The goal of most research is to explain all of the variance among or between variables. This goal is rarely achieved because of the complexity of man and human behavior. However, in this study a reasonable amount of variance (42 percent) was explained by these two sets of variables. This provides researchers with a logical and empirical direction for continued exploration.

DISCUSSION AND RECOMMENDATIONS

It has been demonstrated in this study that there are at least two dimensions that account for the relationship between human synergistic development and human field motion. These dimensions are most likely the independent relational properties of unitary man's development. The variables in each set that were used to measure these properties contribute to each dimension and by definition provide each with a description.

Secondly, we can ponder from the results the nature of the relationship (Tables 9–1 and 9–2). Creativity traits, differentiation, and six evaluative and/or potency human field motion scales contribute to the first canonical variate. Because differentiation is a stable characteristic and because there is an equal distribution of scales on both concepts reflecting human field motion, it appears that a diverse pattern and organization may be accounted for by this dimension. Also, the loadings on these canonical variables, which are similar to factors, are not consistently

TABLE 9–1. VARIABLES CONTRIBUTING TO THE FIRST DIMENSION (N = 213)

Canonical Correlation = 0.41*
Eigenvalue = 0.17

Variable set	Complexity-diversity pattern Canonical variate 1	
Human field motion	*My motor is running*	
	Weak–strong	−0.42[†]
	Drag–propel	0.51
	Sleepy–wakeful	−0.43
	My field expansion	
	Dark–bright	−0.44
	Finite–boundaryless	−0.45
	Dull–sharp	0.68
Human synergistic development	Creativity traits	0.94
	Differentiation	−0.37

*p = 0.001
[†]Weights considered relevant above 0.35 based upon the formula:
$(1/\sqrt{N-IV-DV}) \times$ standard error $= (1/\sqrt{213-20}) \times 5 = 0.35$[19]

TABLE 9–2. VARIABLES CONTRIBUTING TO THE SECOND DIMENSION (N = 213)

Canonical Correlation = 0.37*
Eigenvalue = 0.14

Variable set	Human field motion Canonical variate 2	
Human field motion	*My motor is running* Dull–sharp	0.37[†]
	My field expansion Discontinuous–continuous	0.47
	Pragmatic–visionary	−0.41
	Passive–active	0.72
	Cowardly–brave	−0.40
	Weak–strong	−0.66
Human synergistic development	Time experience	0.90

*p = 0.01
†Weights considered relevant above 0.35 based upon the formula:
$(1/\sqrt{N-IV-DV}) \times$ standard error $= (1/\sqrt{213-20}) \times 5 = 0.35$[19]

in the same direction as when the human field motion tool is factored alone. The principle of helicy can account for this complexity.

The variable contribution to the second canonical variate are five scales rated on the field expansion concept, one scale of "my motor is running," and time experience. This dimension has variables contributing that are related to space and temporal concepts. Although there may be confusion to the name given this dimension, it most likely is the "experiential multidimensional position" that is proposed to be human field motion.

Thus, the Human Field Motion Tool is probably a measure of more than human field motion. It may also be a measure of slower changing pattern and organization evidenced by this first canonical variate. There may be two dimensions that evolve at differing perceptual rates of change, and the change may be relative to other conditions.

Rogers[27] has postulated that human development is "dynamic, multidimensional, synergistic and negentropic . . . and is characterized by increasing complexity and diversity of energy field pattern and organization." Through this study we have seen that this is so. The complexity–diversity pattern, although characterizing all human fields, probably differs uniquely for individuals. If we could investigate the variable patterns as they occur thematically and perhaps temporally, we might begin to understand the nature of this human synergistic development.

It is proposed that the dimension termed complexity–diversity pattern is, through our current measurement and perception, a slower changing characteristic than is the second dimension of human field motion. It is proposed that human field motion is a characteristic of development that contributes to an identifiable pattern and organization and accounts for a space–time coordinate essential in the synthesis of four-dimensional energy fields. It is proposed that human field motion is an alternative to temporality and spatial variables and that the latter two will not directly help to specify the phenomena of unitary man or his evolution.

The following recommendations, many of which are challenging, are all risk-taking and must be viewed within the language and framework of Science of Unitary Man:

- Examine the Human Field Motion Tool for retest stability in light of the discussion that some scales may change at different rates and relative to other variable changes
- Develop additional instruments for measuring human field motion to facilitate construct validation and raise questions of the nature of change
- Consider human field motion as an alternative to time experience in the study of synergistic human development
- Investigate the relationship between physical motion and human field motion

Lastly, regardless of how one chooses to investigate man's development, it is imperative to use consistency with a selected, guiding theoretical framework. In the interest of nursing science, the phenomena of study must be able to be specified, and theories must be derived to enable explanation and perhaps prediction of man's development. Rogers has provided nursing with a conceptual system for viewing unitary man. This author has chosen to empirically investigate man's development through this view and foresees that many will add to the empirical validation of this nursing science.

REFERENCES

1. Barron F: Creativity and Personal Freedom. Princeton, Van Nostrand, 1968
2. Bassili J, Farber J: Experiments on the locus of induced motion. Percep Psychophys 21:157–61, 1977
3. Bondy NK: An Investigation through Semantic Encoding of the Differences in Selected Environmental Events by Varying Shape and Motion, doctoral dissertation. New York University, 1975 (University Microfilms)
4. Braunstein ML: Minimal conditions for perception of rotary motion. Scand J Psychol 18:216–223, 1977
5. Capra F: The Tao of Physics. Berkeley, Shambala, 1975
6. Cohen J, Cohen P: Applied Multiple Regresson/Correlation Analysis for the Behavioral Sciences. New York, Wiley, 1975
7. DelGaudio A: Psychological differentiation and mobility as related to creativity. Percept Mot Skills 43:831–841, 1976
8. Domino G: Identification of potentially creative persons from the adjective check list. J Consult Clin Psychol 35:48–51, 1970
9. Dubin R: Theory Building. New York, Free Press, 1969
10. Edge HL: Personal survival and the meaning of life. American Society for Psychical Research Newsletter 4(3):1–2, 1978

11. Earle A: The Effect of Supplementary Postnatal Kinesthetic Stimulation on the Developmental Behavior of the Normal Female Newborn, doctoral dissertation. New York University, 1969 (University Microfilms)
12. Favreau OE: Interference in colour ontingent motion aftereffects. Q J Exp Psychol 28:553–560, 1978
13. Ference HM: The Relationship of Time Experience, Creativity Traits, Differentiation, and Human Field Motion: An Empirical Investigation of Rogers' Correlates of Synergistic Human Development, doctoral dissertation. New York University, 1979 (University Microfilms)
14. Gough HG, Heilbrun AB: The Adjective Check List Manual. Palo Alto, Consulting Psychologists Press, 1965
15. Knapp RH, Garbutt JT: Time imagery and achievement motive. J Pers 26:421–434, 1958
16. Kolers P: Aspects of Motion Perception. New York, Pergamon Press, 1972
17. May R: The Courage to Create. New York, Norton, 1975
18. Maslow AH: Toward a Psychology of Being, 2nd ed. Princeton, Van Nostrand, 1968
19. Merrifield P: Factor, varieties of description and confirmation. Lecture presented at New York University, November 14, 1978
20. Neal M: The Relationship Between a Regimen of Vestibular Stimulation and Developmental Behavior of the Small Premature Infant, doctoral dissertation. New York University, 1967
21. Nunnally JC: Psychometric Theory. New York, McGraw-Hill, 1967
22. Oppenheimer JR: The need for new knowledge. In Wolfle D (ed): Symposium on Basic Research. Washington, D.C., American Association for the Advancement of Science, 1959
23. Osgood CE, Suci GJ: Factor analysis of meaning. J Exp Psychol 50:325–338, 1955
24. Osgood CE, Suci GJ, Tannenbaum PH: The Measurement of Meaning. Chicago, University of Illinois Press, 1957
25. Porter L: Physical-Physiological Activity and Infants' Growth and Development, doctoral dissertation. New York University, 1967 (University Microfilms)
26. Rogers ME: Nursing Science: A science of unitary man, terminology. New York University, September 10, 1978 (unpublished)
27. Rogers ME: Postulated correlates of unitary human development. New York University, September, 1977 (unpublished)
28. Rogers ME: An Introduction to the Theoretical Basis of Nursing. Philadelphia, F.A. Davis, 1970
29. Rogers ME, Ference H, Winstead-Fry P: Personal conferences on science of unitary man. New York University, Fall 1979
30. Schmeidler G, Windholz G: A nonverbal indicator of attitude. J Cross-Cult Psych 3(4):383–394, 1972
31. Smith JM, Schaefer CE: Development of a creativity scale for the adjective check list. Psychol Rep 25:87–92, 1969
32. Snider, Osgood CE (eds): Appendix: Semantic Atlas of 550 Concepts: Semantic Differential Techniques. Chicago, Aldine, 1975
33. Torgerson W: Theory and Methods of Scaling. New York, Wiley, 1958
34. Wallach MA, Green LR: On age and the subjective speed of time. J Gerontol 16:71–74, 1961
35. Webster's 7th New Collegiate Dictionary. Springfield, Mass, Merriam, 1963
36. Witkin H, Goodenough E, Oltman P: Psychological Differentiation: Current Status. Princeton, Educational Testing Services, 1977 (Research Bulletin No. 77–17)

37. Witkin HA, Oltman PK, Raskin E, Karp SA: Embedded Figures Test Manual. Palo Alto, Consulting Psychologists Press, 1971
38. Yonge GD: Time experiences, self-actualizing values, and creativity. J Pers Assess 39:601–606, 1975
39. Zukav G: The Dancing Wu Li Masters: An Overview of the New Physics. New York, Morrow, 1979

Critique of Ference's Study

Joyce J. Fitzpatrick

Rogers' principle of resonancy served as the major guiding force for this study. Ference postulated four indices, including human field motion, creativity, differentiation, and time experience, developed from Rogers' conceptualizations regarding synergistic humans. While some general conceptual links were presented well by Ference, there continues to be a need for more depth in the conceptual argument. And, importantly, theoretical links could be provided; they would greatly enhance the investigation. What is especially needed is a deeper explication of the concept of motion to support the evaluative statements.

An important contribution of this research was development and testing of the Human Field Motion Tool, which was then used in subsequent research. Ference presented some information regarding the instrument development. But the serious student of Rogers desires every detail, so that such instrument construction and evaluation can be expanded. The lack of available instruments to measure holistic concepts has long been a concern in relation to research based on Rogers' model. It is hoped that the evaluation of this instrument will continue, and that the instrument can be refined. Psychometric assessment of the instrument as presented here warrants further evaluation.

Another methodological aspect of this study that was only minimally addressed was the set of instruments used to measure human field development. These instruments were developed from different conceptualizations, and Ference assumed conceptual fit. Further validity testing would be desired to ascertain more fully the relationship to Rogers' conceptualizations. This theoretical and empirical assessment could provide the subject for many subsequent studies.

Ference discussed both the conceptual and methodological limitations of the variable set in relation to her results. The discussion of results that she presented was most enlightening in relation to further clarification of research in this area. Most significant was the statement that the Human Field Motion Tool was probably a measure of more than human field motion. Ference's speculations here were challenging. One could be enticed to continue this line of investigation in order to clarify the proposed relationships. Various questions regarding future conceptualizations were posed by the results of this research. Of particular interest was the extent to which there is overlap in some of the major concepts proposed by Rogers. It remains for future researchers to clarify pattern and organization, diversity and complexity, and field motion and development. A recommendation for conceptual, theoretical, and subsequent empirical clarification is made.

As reflected in Ference's recommendations for future research, this investigation was viewed as a beginning, an exploratory attempt to explicate key relationships postulated by Rogers. It is important that future researchers continue to attend to the need for clarification and refinement. Each future study should reflect analysis based on this early work of Ference. Thus, it would be possible to accumulate considerable data that could then be used for further instrument evaluation and development.

As was proposed here, there is a continued need for further continued clarification of conceptual and empirical links. It is anticipated that such study will be enlightened by this work of Ference.

Response

Helen M. Ference

The purpose of this chapter is to provide a brief overview of a major theoretical construct, its tool development, pilot testing, and the empirical testing of 213 subjects. The serious student is encouraged to read the complete study, under the same title, published through University Microfilms (No. 80–10, 281). The conceptual and logical arguments for selecting the indices of human synergistic development are presented in that final report. Additionally, the Human Field Motion Tool is presented with the psychometric and statistical justification for its reliability and validity.

The instruments were not assumed to have conceptual fit, as inferred by Fitzpatrick. Rather, three instruments were logically revalidated as measures of human synergistic development, and one tool was specifically developed for first-time use as a measure of the four-dimensional human energy field. This first-time measure, the Human Field Motion Tool, was specifically developed to measure motion as an index of human synergistic development. It was the first tool reported in the literature that was solely developed as a measure in the Science of Unitary Human Beings (Man). The three other tools used—the Time Metaphor Test, the Adjective Check List, and the Group Embedded Figures Test—were logically revalidated as measures of time experience, creativity and differentiation, as theoretically defined according to the Science of Unitary Human Beings.

10

The Relationship Between Hyperactivity in Children and Perception of Short Wavelength Light

Violet M. Malinski

This theoretical research was undertaken as an initial exploration of hyperactivity within the Science of Unitary Human Beings proposed for nursing by Rogers. The investigator selected Rogers' theory of accelerating evolution within which to test for possible correlations between hyperactivity and perception of short wavelength light. Because "perception" is global in nature, two measurable components were isolated: vision along the short wavelength end of the spectrum and expressed color preferences. Data were collected on 104 boys aged 8 through 12. Hyperactivity was assessed according to 19 behavioral items on a scale compiled by a private child development institute that offers nutritional and sensorimotor therapies for hyperactive children. A correlational design was used to test the hypotheses predicting relationships among hyperactivity, perception of short wavelength light, and preference for hues associated with the shorter wavelengths of light. Neither hypothesis received statistical support.

BACKGROUND: GENESIS OF PROBLEM FORMULATION

Despite intensive study by members of varied professions focusing on a range of variables, the phenomenon commonly labeled "hyperactivity" is not understood completely. Etiological theories and treatment approaches vary, as do descriptions of the clinical picture presented. There is a growing body of research to support the idea that "hyperactivity is a non-specific symptom occurring in a variety of medical and behavioral disorders and associated with a heterogenous group of etiological factors."[38] My experiences in child and adolescent psychiatric nursing highlighted the confusion and difficulties encountered by the family when a child entered the medical treatment system with such a diagnosis. Having worked as a public health nurse in a school, I knew firsthand the dilemmas posed by being the person designated to dispense prescribed medications, such as Ritalin, to school children and was, therefore, eager to explore a different framework for understanding such children and the alternative treatment approaches such a framework might generate.

Hyperactivity

Some 40 labels have been coined to describe children, usually boys aged 5 through 12, given such a diagnosis. Postulated etiological theories range from deficits in attention and motivation[1, 9, 16] to diencephalic dysfunction resulting in cortical overstimulation[22] to understimulation resulting from lowered central nervous system arousal levels[40] or insufficient sensory stimulation[48] to allergic reactions to artificial food flavors and dyes[14] to psychogenic factors such as childrearing practices.

One common assumption is that some type of organic dysfunction is operating in a majority of cases. After reviewing studies in this area, Dubey[13] concluded that evidence to support this is minimal. Studies have also failed to find correlations among symptoms, suggesting a great degree of heterogeneity among the children and casting doubt on the existence of a discrete syndrome.[7, 42]

Light

It has been suggested that light is the synchronizer of fundamental biochemical and hormonal rhythms in some living systems.[15, 23–25, 45] Light plays a role in neuroendocrine functions such as onset of pubescence[45, 46] and ovulation.[12, 26] Light penetrates deeply into mammalian tissue, passing through the skull and reaching the brain directly.[43, 45] Living systems also contain a variety of pigments capable of photoreactions.[20] It is postulated that light affects development of the pineal gland from birth, possibly accelerating its development.[26] Living systems, therefore, do not need to see light to interact with it.

Wurtman and Neer[47] and Ott[32] have recommended that the spectral distributions of standard artificial light be readjusted to approximate that of natural sunlight. Such a change would incorporate, for example, the near ultraviolet portion of the spectrum. Mayron, Ott, Nations, and Mayron[29, 30] conducted experiments in public schools designed to test the effects of standard fluorescent lights compared with full-spectrum lights, which more closely approximate the spectral distribution of sunlight, on hyperactive behaviors, maintaining that the children under the full spectrum lighting showed a decrease in hyperactive behaviors.

Zentall and Zentall[49] recommend the use for hyperactive children of multistimuli learning centers incorporating lights, bright colors, and music. They postulated that hyperactive children suffer from "sensory blocking or overfiltering" for which the high level of environmental stimuli compensates.[49]

Perhaps another way to look at such studies is to consider the hyperactive child as a manifestation of growing diversity and accelerated field rhythms. In an effort to explore this avenue of thinking, the following problem question was posed: What is the relationship of hyperactivity in children, perception of short wavelength light, and color preferences?

RELATIONSHIP TO THE SCIENCE OF UNITARY HUMAN BEINGS

Conceptual systems have the capacity to generate numerous theories. One which Rogers has developed is the theory of accelerating evolution, according to which "change is postulated to proceed in the direction of higher wave frequency field pattern and of organization characterized by growing diversity."[37]

Human and environment are continually evolving together via their continuous, mutual process of interaction. This is Rogers' principle of complementarity. The principle of helicy describes the nature and direction of this development as creative and innovative, manifesting increasing diversity and complexity of field pattern. According to the principle of resonancy, the human and environmental fields are identified by pattern, perceived as a mosaic of waves, and manifesting continuous change from longer waves of lower frequencies toward shorter waves of higher frequencies.

Wavelength and frequency are related to the diversity and complexity of pattern, with the shift toward shorter wavelengths associated with faster rhythms and accelerating evolutionary development. Rogers has postulated dynamic, nonlinear correlates of the nature and direction of change in unitary human beings, noting that change is relative and in constant flux (see Chapter 2). Those specific to the study are:

Change from	In the Direction of	
Lower frequency patterns	Higher frequency patterns	Seem continuous
Longer rhythms	Shorter rhythms	Seem continuous
Slower motion	Faster motion	Seem continuous

Within this continuum, the hyperactive child is postulated to be on the evolving edge. Thus, he or she would be expected to show indications of faster rhythms, increased motion, and other behaviors indicative of this shift toward resonating wave patterns of increasing velocity and energy.

Light is a wave, a "vibrational pattern."[8] The color spectrum of visible light ranges from long wave low frequency (red) through short wave high frequency (violet) spectral hues. Because wavelength is inversely proportional to momentum, the shorter the wavelength the higher the momentum. Energy is proportional to frequency. Therefore, violet light, with a short wavelength and high frequency, has a high degree of momentum and energy, whereas red light, with a long wavelength and low frequency, has low momentum and energy.[8]

If the hyperactive child, as postulated, is a manifestation of accelerating rhythms, has he or she evolved further in the direction of higher frequency patterns of light than children perceived as "normal"? Would this be manifested with perception of numbers illuminated in a field of short wavelength light and with color preferences among spectral hues associated with long and short wavelength light?

METHOD

After consultation with my committee, I decided to use a rating scale as an objective measure of hyperactivity. In order to provide a wide range of ratings on the hyperactivity scale to correlate with any differences observed in the wave phenomena of light and color under study, a volunteer sample of 104 boys, aged 8 through 12, was obtained from a private treatment center that utilizes nutritional and sensorimotor therapies as an alternative to drug therapy and from four private schools, all in the same city. No child was selected who had a diagnosis of dyslexia or brain injury.

A written explanation was provided to the parent(s). I answered any questions and assured them that their children could withdraw at any time. Once written consent was obtained, I met with the child, provided a simplified written explanation, assured him that he was free to stop at any time, answered any questions, and obtained the child's written consent.

The rating scale for hyperactivity had been in use at the institute for 5 years. The investigator analyzed it for reliability, interrater reliability, and discriminant ability. For item reliability, Cronbach alphas were obtained of 0.92 (mothers), 0.93 (fathers), and 0.96 (teachers). Interrater reliabilities were obtained of 0.83 (mother–father–teacher), 0.70 (mother–father), 0.70 (mother–teacher), and 0.58 (father–teacher). Each subject was rated by at least one parent and teacher. The average of the ratings was computed and recorded as the hyperactivity score for each child.

Discriminant function analysis was used to assess the ability of the scale to distinguish diagnosed and nondiagnosed groups. A discriminant function is a regression equation utilizing group membership as the dependent variable.[19] Of the 104 cases, 85 percent were considered to be correctly classified.

In order to rule out color-blind subjects, the investigator used the American Optical Company Pseudoisochromatic Plates, a valid tool in detecting the two primary types of color blindness, blue-yellow and red-green.[6] The color samples, obtained from the Munsell Color Company, were calibrated according to the three dimensions of hue, value (brightness), and chroma (saturation). Because hue was the dimension under study, value and chroma were controlled at middle levels, 6 and 8 respectively. Hue level was controlled at 5. Therefore, the Munsell color notation for each sample was represented by 5 (hue letter) 6/8. The wavelength equivalents for each spectral hue follow, given in nanometers (nm).

Hue	Wavelength	Hue	Wavelength
5R6/8	607	5G6/8	513
5YR6/8	587.5	5BG6/8	493
5Y6/8	577	5B6/8	484.5
5GY6/8	566	5PB6/8	476

Because most artificial samples of violet are compounds of blue and red, the wavelength equivalents fall in the middle of the 500-nm range rather than toward 400 nm, the area where visible light is perceived as violet. Therefore, no violet sample was included.

The light-emitting device used in the vision test was the S. C. Colorimeter, produced by Technicon Corporation. Seven pairs of narrow-band transmission filters (Technicon) were used to graduate the wavelength of light in the following steps: 480, 440, 400, 375, 367, 352, and 340 nm. Because brightness of light was proportional to filter wavelength, Kodak Wratten Neutral Density Filters were used to hold brightness constant. They were calibrated on a log function against the dimmest filter, 340 nm. The appropriate neutral density filter was used in conjunction with each of the narrow-band transmission filters. Because of the extremely low levels of ambient light to be measured, a 610 BR Electrometer, produced by Keithley Instruments, was used in conjunction with an EG & G Silicon Photodiode UV-100 to measure the amount of light in the darkened rooms.

Because each participating facility requested that its children be tested on their premises, different settings were used and efforts made to assure comparable environmental conditions. I conducted the vision test in a dark-green, self-supporting, portable tent in order to minimize differences due to environment. In the darkened rooms of each facility, readings were obtained of 0.01×10^{-11} amperes, or about 1/20th of the ambient light in a typically illuminated room, before vision testing began.

If the potential subject passed the test for color blindness, he was given the color preference test. Eight 8 1/2 × 11-inch black matte cards on which the Munsell color samples (3 × 5 inches) had been mounted were presented with instructions to order them from most to least preferred colors. Because the testing rooms had different natural exposures, the subject looked at the samples under a lamp having a color temperature of 7500° Kelvin, the Color-Classer produced by Duro-Test Corporation.

Because the dark-adapted eye is maximally sensitive to shorter wavelengths, the child was dark-adapted for 5 minutes before the vision test began. I then illuminated a sample test card. With the first pair of filters in place, I instructed the child to sit at a distance where he could discern and identify the number on the card. He was then instructed not to shift position, guess at a number, or strain his eyes. For each pair of filters inserted in the prescribed sequence, I held a black matte card, 3 × 1 inches, imprinted with a number in white ink approximately 1/4-inch high, about 6 inches from the light source and asked the child to read the number. If he correctly identified the number, I inserted the next pair of filters. If he did not, I stopped and turned on the lights.

RESULTS

A correlational design was employed with the independent variable, hyperactivity, on a continuum of possible scores ranging from 0 through 57. The first dependent variable was the last filter wavelength under which the child correctly identified the illuminated number. By means of the *Statistical Packages for the Social Sciences,*[31] a scattergram was plotted and a Pearson r computed to test the relationship between hyperactivity and vision along the short wavelength end of the spectrum. Although the obtained r of -0.11 fell in the predicted direction, this result was not significant at the 0.05 level.

Because a trend toward preference for short wavelength colors was the factor under considertion in the ranking of the eight color choices, each subject's first four choices were recoded according to the number of short wavelength colors present (G, BG, B, PB). The hypothesis was then subjected to regression analysis for one continuous (hyperactivity) and one categorical variable (color preferences). Although in the predicted direction, the obtained rs were not significant. Supplemental analysis was performed with rank order correlation; none of the computed Spearman rs met the criterion of significance at 0.05.

DISCUSSION AND RECOMMENDATIONS

Because the independent variable of hyperactivity was operationalized as a continuous measure, the subjects were not dichotomized into hyperactive and nonhyperactive groups for the purpose of data analysis. The mean for the 104 subjects was 436.9 nm, with a mode of 440 nm. However, if the institute children and school children are examined separately, the former have a lower mean, 429.3 as opposed to 444.4, although both have the same mode of 440. Four of the institute children correctly identified numbers illuminated with the 340 filter, whereas none of the school children were able to do so. The lowest filter at which any of these children correctly identified the illuminated number was 375. It might prove fruitful to administer the vision test first, identify those children with readings below 400 nm, and then examine them in relation to the hyperactivity variable.

The field illuminated by the spectrometer was relatively small, necessitating that the figures on the cards be only 1/4 inch high in order to be completely illuminated. Another type of instrument with a larger field could be used in future studies, perhaps ameliorating possible confusion over numbers such as "3" and "8," which could be mistaken for one another. It is also possible that some subjects told the investigator they could not see the numbers, knowing that she would then turn on the lights.

Some children appeared uncomfortable in the darkened room. Because this had been noted during an earlier pilot study, the investigator dark-adapted the subjects for a 5-minute period only, following preadaptation to a white background, as advised by a consultant. For adults, it takes an average of 40 minutes of dark adaptation before the rods become maximally sensitive to light.[18] Better results might be anticipated with a longer period of dark adaptation.

Although operational definition and measurement are critical to the type of investigation undertaken, the difficulties associated with defining and measuring hyperactivity are well documented. Prevalence rates differ when framed within medical and educational perspectives. Among elementary school children, psychiatric estimates of incidence range from 4 to 10 percent whereas educators place it as high as 15 to 20 percent.[17] When parents, teachers, and physicians were asked to identify hyperactive children in a sample of 5,000 elementary school pupils, 5 percent were rated as such by at least one source, whereas only 1.19 percent were so rated by all three.[21]

There is a lack of developmental norms for such descriptors as activity level. Based on a longitudinal study begun in 1956, Thomas, Chess, and Birch[41] identified a high level of activity as a normal pattern for some children. Activity was only one of nine characteristics of rhythmic patterning identified.

Various rating scales have been proposed and problems identified, as well as mechanical devices for measurement, such as actometers and pedometers, worn on wrist and ankle respectively, to record movement. Correlations among such measures are questionable.[2, 10]

A methodological study could be undertaken for the purpose of developing a measuring tool that can be administered directly to the child, thus providing a hyperactivity profile according to the child's own responses. Such a test could take the form of a semantic differential or metaphor test developed with concepts involving wave correlates of unitary development, including motion, time perception, and differentiation. Posing the question, "What color do you feel like?" is an alternative to "What color do you prefer?" A high frequency environmental field characterized by, for example, high frequency colors, full spectrum light, and music could be organized with filmed records made of children's behaviors in this setting over time. Perhaps what is perceived as a short attention span for some children might indicate a faster pace of learning.

The subjects showed an overall preference for colors associated with the shorter wavelengths, with 62.5 percent choosing three to four such colors among their first four choices. This result is especially interesting in view of the fact that individual color vision is most variable along this portion of the spectrum[11] and blue-violet deficiencies have been noted in children.[27, 28] The investigator noted that a number of children had difficulty discriminating between the B and PB color samples. Their typical comment was, "These are the same color."

Such observations are of particular interest in view of support for the perceptual evolution of color vision from long toward short wavelengths.[5, 36, 39, 44] Despite the apparent difficulty and variability of visual discrimination along this portion of the spectrum, subjects frequently chose these colors, which further supports the conclusion that visual perception of light is only a small part of a holistic interaction.

Color preference, therefore, may not be the most appropriate method to examine the process under consideration. Birren,[3] for example, noted the difference between responses to a color when it appears on the walls of a room as opposed to a colored light that totally saturates the environment. Looking at samples of particular colors is an objective experience, remaining external. It is conceivable that research into human and environmental field interaction with variables of light and color may be best undertaken where light of different wavelengths can be altered.

Although lack of support for the hypotheses may be due to methodology rather than theory, the possibility that the theory is incorrect with respect to the postulated relationships must be acknowledged. Within the model of unitary human beings, human and environment continually evolve via the principle of complementarity, the continual, mutual process toward increasing complexity and diversity of field pattern and organization. This process is emergent evolution. Although their approaches are based on different world views, other researchers and theoreticians are exploring consonant ideas.

In 1977 Prigogine[35] won the Nobel Prize for chemistry for his theory of dissipative structures (dynamic states), which highlights this process of emergence. Prigogine's research suggests that the Second Law of Thermodynamics—that everything is running down or increasing in entropy—does not hold true for some open systems, which dissipate the entropy into the environment with which they interact, thus running up or increasing in complexity, moving toward further evolution rather than gradual decay. He views humans as well as total cultures as examples of such dissipative structures, interacting with probabilistic, nonlinear forces.

The dynamic nature of dissipative structures may provide a possible link to the holonomic model proposed by physicist Bohm and the holographic model by neuroscientist Pribram. Holonomy is the law of the whole. According to Bohm,[4] relativity and quantum theories imply undivided wholeness, whereby analysis of parts becomes irrelevant. Pribram[34] postulated that all perception occurs in the frequency domain, with the brain processing this information to construct images that fit three-dimensional perception.

"Frequency domain" is what Bohm calls the implicate order in his formulation of a holonomic universe where everything is present at once. Each individual is in total contact with this implicate order, which is made explicate by a process of unfolding or holomovement. Prigogine's theory of dissipative structures may be convergent with this explicate or unfolding process.

Pribram's[33, 34] studies led him to the importance of wave phenomena. Bohm's[4] work supports the boundaryless quality of human and environment interaction. Prigogine[35] is exploring the emergence of more complex and diverse forms.

The bases of the conceptual system of unitary human development are energy fields, pattern, open systems, and four-dimensionality. Explorations within this holistic framework must move beyond study of discrete parts with extrapolation to the whole, which was not achieved in the present study. The focus of nursing is unitary human development in the continuing mutual interaction with the environment. By focusing on this process as a holistic unit rather than a dichotomy, the nurse can assist individuals in identifying their own rhythms and activating those potentials that offer maximum well-being. Strategies are needed that promote more harmonious interaction. These can be evolved as we gain in understanding the potentials for change as the human and environmental fields interact, specifically in the area of wave phenomena. The data generated may continuously shape nursing theory and practice as the human field engages in endless repatterning in the dynamic process of becoming.

REFERENCES

1. Anderson RP, Halcomb CG, Doyle RB: The measurement of attentional deficits. Except Child 39:534–538, 1973
2. Barkley RA, Ullman DG: A comparison of objective measures of activity and distractibility in hyperactive and nonhyperactive children. J Abnorm Child Psychol 3:231–234, 1975
3. Birren F: Color Psychology and Color Therapy. New York, University Books, 1961
4. Bohm D: Wholeness and the Implicate Order. Boston, Routledge & Kegan Paul, 1980
5. Bucke RM: Cosmic Consciousness. New York, Dutton, 1973 (Originally published 1901)
6. Burnham RW, Hanes RM, Bartleson CJ: Color: A Guide to Basic Facts and Concepts. New York, Wiley, 1973
7. Campbell S: Hyperactivity: Course and treatment. In Davids A (ed): Child Personality and Psychopathology: Current Topics, Vol 3. New York, Wiley, 1976
8. Capra F: The Tao of Physics. Berkeley, Shamhala, 1975
9. Conners CK, Eisenberg L, Barcai A: Effect of dextroamphetamine on children. Arch Gen Psychiatry 17:478–485, 1967
10. Cromwell RL, Baumeister A, Hawkins WF: Research in activity level. In Ellis NR (ed): Handbook of Mental Deficiency. New York, McGraw-Hill, 1963
11. Davidoff JB: Differences in Visual Perception. New York, Academic Press, 1975
12. Dewan E: On the possibility of a perfect rhythm method of birth control by periodic light stimulation. Am J Obstet Gynecol 99:1016–1019, 1967
13. Dubey DR: Organic factors in hyperkinesis: A critical evaluation. Am J Orthopsychiatry 46:353–366, 1976
14. Feingold BG: Hyperkinesis and learning disabilities linked to artificial food flavors and colors. Am J Nurs 75:797–803, 1975
15. Gerritzen F: Influence of light on human circadian rhythms. Aerospace Med 37:66–70, 1966
16. Greenberg IM, Deem MA, McMahon S: Effects of dextroamphetamine, chlorpromazine, and hydroxyzine on behavior and performance in hyperactive children. Am J Psychiatry 129:532–539, 1972
17. Grinspoon L, Singer S: Amphetamines in the treatment of hyperkinetic children. In Chess S, Thomas A (eds): Annual Progress in Child Psychiatry and Child Development. New York, Brunner/Mazel, 1975, pp 417–456
18. Kaufman L: Sight and Mind. New York, Oxford University Press, 1974
19. Kerlinger FN, Pedhazur EJ: Multiple Regression in Behavioral Research. New York, Holt, Rinehart & Winston, 1973
20. Klein R: Shedding light on the use of light. Pediatrics 50:118–126, 1972
21. Lambert NM, Sandoval J, Sassone D: Prevalence of hyperactivity in elementary school

children as a function of social system definers. Am J Orthopsychiatry 48:446–463, 1978

22. Laufer M, Denhoff E, Solomons G: Hyperkinetic impulse disorder in children's behavior problems. Psychosom Med 19:38–48, 1957

23. Loban M, Tedre B: Renal diurnal rhythms in an arctic mining community. J Physiol (London) 165:75P–76P, 1963

24. Loban M, Tedre B: Renal diurnal rhythms in blind subjects. J Physiol (London) 170:29P–30P, 1964

25. Loban M., Tedre B: Perception of light and the maintenance of renal diurnal rhythms. J Physiol (London) 189:32–33, 1961

26. Luce GG: Body Time. New York, Pantheon, 1971

27. MacCambridge SW: Efficiency of Color Combinations on Perception of Educationally Handicapped and Noneducationally Handicapped Children, doctoral dissertation. University of North Colorado, 1974. (Dissertation Abstracts International, 1975, 35:5972A, University Microfilms No. 75–5425)

28. McGraw-Hill. Schools blind to vision problems. Nation's Schools Report, November 24, 1975, 1–2

29. Mayron LW, Ott J, Nations R, Mayron EL: Light, radiation, and academic behavior. Acad Ther Quart 10:33–47, 1974

30. Mayron LW, Mayron E, Ott J, Nations, R: Light radiation and academic achievement: Second-year data. Acad Ther Quart 11:397–407, 1976

31. Nie NH, Hull CH, Jenkins JH, Steinbrenner K, Brent DH: Statistical Package for the Social Sciences, 2nd ed. New York, McGraw-Hill, 1975

32. Ott JN: Health and Light. Old Greenwich, Conn, Devin-Adair, 1973

33. Pribram KH: Languages of the Brain. Monterey, Calif, Brooks/Cole, 1971

34. Pribram KH: What the fuss is all about. ReVision 1:14–18, 1978

35. Prigogine I: From Being to Becoming: Time and Complexity in the Physical Sciences. San Francisco, W. H. Freeman, 1980

36. Robertson PW: Colour words and colour vision. Bio Human Affairs 33:28–33, 1967

37. Rogers ME: Nursing: A science of unitary man. In Riehl JP, Roy C (eds): Conceptual Models for Nursing Practice, 2nd ed. New York, Appleton-Century-Crofts, 1980

38. Ross DM, Ross SA: Hyperactivity Research Theory Action. New York, Wiley, 1976

39. Sahlins M: Colors and cultures. Semiotica 16:1–22, 1976

40. Satterfield JH, Dawson M: Electrodermal correlates of hyperactivity in children. Psychophysiology 8:191–197, 1971

41. Thomas A, Chess S, Birth H: Temperament and Behavior Disorders in Children. New York, New York University Press, 1968

42. Ullman DG, Barkley RA, Brown HW: The behavior symptoms of hyperkinetic children who successfully responded to stimulant drug treatment. Am J Orthopsychiatry 48:425–437, 1978

43. van Brunt EE, Sheperd MD, Wall JR, Ganong WF, Clegg MT: Penetration of light into the brain of mammals. Ann NY Acad Sci 117:217–227, 1964

44. Werner H: Comparative Psychology of Mental Development. New York, International Universities Press, 1948

45. Wurtman R: The effects of light on the human body. Sci Am 233:69–77, 1975

46. Wurtman R, Weisel J: Environmental lighting and neuroendocrine function: Relationship between spectrum of light source and gonadal growth. Endocrinology 85:1218–1221, 1969

47. Wurtman R, Neer RM: Good light and bad. N Engl J Med 282:394–395, 1970

48. Zentall S: Optimal stimulation as theoretical basis of hyperactivity. Am J Orthopsychiatry 45:549–561, 1975
49. Zentall S, Zentall T: Activity and task performance of hyperactive children as a function of environmental stimulation. J Consult Clin Psychol 44:693–696, 1976

Critique of Malinski's Study

Joyce J. Fitzpatrick

Malinski was concerned with the relationship between hyperactivity and perception of short wavelength light. While many researchers relate their studies to Rogers' broad principles, Malinski has appropriately narrowed her interest to a specific set of relationships posited by Rogers in a theory of accelerating evolution. This is clearly a strength of Malinski's study. What remains unclear, however, is the specific theoretical propositions that are delineated by this theory. For example, it is not specified how this particular theory is related to Rogers' assumptions and principles; much must be inferred. Such inferences are only possible if the reader is familiar with Rogers' conceptualization.

Another strength of Malinski's work is the direct relationship to a behavioral manifestation—hyperactivity—that has been of interest to nurses. Such practical relevance has been requested by nurses who are confronted with the day-to-day problems of helping persons achieve health.

Malinski seemed to be well aware of the major problems with this study. A significant problem was the operationalization of the independent variable, hyperactivity. The author noted the amorphous nature of the variable and tried to refine not only the measurement but also the conceptualization. The rating scale for hyperactivity seemed to introduce imprecision into the delineation of this measure. In future research, it is recommended that additional assessments of activity occur so as to more completely attend to concerns of reliability and validity. Observations of activity with simultaneous recordings would be desired. The recommendation that Malinski proposes—that of a child-completed activity assessment—seemed of questional value in relation to the activity variable as defined here. Rather, this change would significantly alter the nature of the study. Thus, perhaps refinement of the conceptualization of hyperactivity as a variable of interest in relation to Rogers' proposed correlate of motion is the highest priority in further development of this research.

The operationalization of the color-perception variable is equally problematic in this study. Quite a limited range of responses is available. More precision in measurement is warranted, again with an effort also placed on clarification of both conceptualization and measurement.

In summary, Malinski's study is clearly an exploratory one. The linking of activity and lightwave variables represents a creative approach to explicating a relationship theoretically derived from Rogers' conceptual model. The author should be challenged to continue the research, focusing the study with a tighter theoretical framework and attention to multiple measurements of key variables.

Response

Violet M. Malinski

In planning a study of hyperactivity within the Science of Unitary Human Beings, I wanted to explore the unitary human field, hypothesizing that the field of a hyperactive child would manifest higher frequency patterning. The difficulty lay in finding a way to do this. I tried to find an analogy to Fourier analysis because Fourier transforms provide a way to convert a finite "thing" into wave patterning distributed throughout space and time. Although I eventually put this idea aside, every now and then I read something that suggests that it is still worth pursuing. (See, for example, Rudolph's discussion of the analogy that he, an applied mathematician, sees between Fourier transforms and LeShan's description of sensory and clairvoyant realities in *The Medium, the Mystic, and the Physicist.*)[1, 2]

I agree with Fitzpatrick's suggestion that refinement of the conceptualization of hyperactivity within this system would be a priority for future research. I recommend that this be done by looking at the experiences, feelings, and perceptions of hyperactive children themselves. The idea for a child-completed hyperactivity assessment tool, for example, also grew out of this idea of exploring patterning of the human field. Items could be designed in line with all the postulated correlates of patterning, not just activity and motion. Within this system, hyperactivity is more than a motion variable, which is why I chose to explore it in relation to wave phenomena operationalized as short wavelength light and colors associated with specific wavelengths along the visible spectrum. Phenomenology, for example, would provide one avenue for exploration of the lived experience of hyperactivity.

REFERENCES

1. LeShan L: The Medium, the Mystic, and the Physicist: Toward a General Theory of the Paranormal. New York, Ballantine Books, 1974
2. Rudolph LD: A speculation on the relationship between LeShan's sensory and clairvoyant realities. ReVision 7:106–112, 1984

11

The Relationship Between Visible Lightwaves and the Experience of Pain

Sharon F. McDonald

This study was intended to determine whether there is a relationship between the human experience of pain and the presence of certain visible lightwaves (colors) in the environment. The rhythm theory component of Martha Rogers' model was used as the conceptual framework. Rhythm theory deals with the human–environment interaction in terms of wave frequencies and patterns. The Principles of Homeodynamics describe these rhythmic relationships. Data were collected from 60 female volunteers between the ages of 40 and 60 years who had a medical diagnosis of rheumatoid arthritis. The study had a mixed experimental design with filter type (red, blue, and control), the presence or absence of a visual barrier, and the duration of exposure as the independent variables. Pre-exposure pain scores were the dependent measures. The first hypothesis dealt with the relationship between the predominant presence of lightwaves and a reduction in pain. Analysis of covariance tests and a multivariate analysis of variance test indicated that subjects exposed to shorter, more frequent lightwaves (blue) were more likely to experience a reduction in pain than were subjects exposed to either the red lightwaves or to a control condition. The barrier variable was shown to be an unimportant factor in the subjects' responses to the filter conditions. The second hypothesis concerned the variable of duration of exposure to lightwaves. Results showed that the longer the exposure to the blue light, the progressively greater the reduction in pain. The results of this study are discussed in terms of their relevance for nursing theory development and professional nursing intervention. Recommendations for replication and modification of the study are discussed.

BACKGROUND: GENESIS OF PROBLEM FORMULATION

One of the primary concerns of nursing is the alleviation of pain. As a community health nurse, I became aware that persons who have the chronic disease of rheumatoid arthritis commonly experience pain of varying degrees as they attempt to carry out their daily activities. These people number into the millions in the United States today.[1] They and the nurses caring for them are actively seeking ways to reduce the pain and discomfort they experience.

The science of nursing is interested in the relationship between variables in the environment and the human responses to health on both theoretical and applied levels. Visible lightwaves are usually known as colors and are one type of environmental variable that may affect an individual's health. People have been involved with colors since the beginning of time. Color has been used as a mode of expression, a protective survival strategy, and as symbolism.[3, 19] As technological methods became available, an analysis of the visible spectrum revealed that the differences among colors lie in the frequency of vibration of the various lightwaves.[8] Violet is the color with the highest vibratory rate, and red has the lowest rate.

In addition to these physical differences, colors are known to have different psychological connotations, which have been found to have universal meaning.[9, 14] Colors have also been shown to be related to a variety of human physiological responses such as blood pressure, galvanic skin response, pulse, and respiration.[4, 5, 16, 19] Many of these studies were conducted with a minimal use of controls and with small samples. However, tentative results suggest that colors do indeed affect the nature of the human being.

RELATIONSHIP TO THE SCIENCE OF UNITARY HUMAN BEINGS

Nursing is concerned with the development of a scientific base of knowledge for the profession. Rogers' conceptual system can guide research efforts in the identification and organization of that knowledge.[18] This study is based on the rhythm theory component of Rogers' model as a framework for describing the relationship between the human experience of pain and the presence of certain visible lightwaves in the environment (Fig. 11–1). The principle of complementarity, as one of the three Principles of Homeodynamics, was the main focus for theory testing in this study. Rogers postulates in the principle of complementarity that human beings and the environment are energy fields that are mutual, inseparable, and continually interacting.[18] Thus, changes in one will be related to changes in the other. If this is really true, then empirically researchers should be able to demonstrate a relationship between a nurse-initiated modification in a person's environment and an alteration in that person's state of being. In this study, the nurse modified the environment by introducing the predominant presence of certain colors and measured possible alterations in the person's pain.

The experience of pain was defined as the self-assessed intensity of overall sensations experienced by the subject, as opposed to the use of one or two physiological or psychological indicators selected by the investigator. This was done to remain consistent with the concept of ''unitary human being'' presented in Rogers' model. A subject's personal assessment of the current pain experience in the presence of these environmental lightwaves was regarded as a manifestation of the

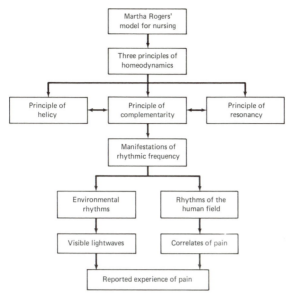

Figure 11–1. Lightwaves and experience of pain: Relationship to Rogers' model.

rhythmic interaction of the person–environment relationship. The amount of pain reported was used as an indicator of that manifestation.

The issue of selection of appropriate indicators to be used as an index of the concept of "unitary human being" needs to be addressed. The assumption used in designing this study was that the experience of pain is a unitary, or whole-person, phenomenon.[10] Pain was selected as the manifestation of field interaction. The appropriateness of this choice is open for discussion. The question arises: Are the correlates of pain true indicators of the human field, and thereby of the concept of unitary human being? To support a positive response to this question, one could argue that the literature describes the concept of pain as a rhythmic phenomenon having wavelike characteristics.[10, 11] Pain has also been described as having two components, the sensory and the reactive, which are influenced by cognitive, social, and cultural variables.[12, 22] This suggests that pain is experienced individually, is broader than any of these factors, and can be regarded as an expression of a person's unitary being.

On the other hand, the use of the experience of pain as a correlate of the human field could be challenged by those who argue that the person's subjective assessment of pain may refer only to a part of the human response rather than to the whole. Since the definition of the concept of pain is left with the subject, there is no assurance that the subject is responding from a sense of wholeness or simply from a fragmented sense of physical, social, or psychological discomfort. In that case the use of correlates of pain could not be considered as an appropriate indicator of the human field or unitary human experience.

METHOD

This study had a mixed experimental design, with filter type, length of time of exposure, and the presence or absence of a visual barrier as the independent variables. Pre-exposure pain scores were obtained before any interventions were undertaken to provide baseline data used as covariates in the analysis. Post-exposure pain scores were the dependent measures.

There were two hypotheses for the study:

1. The predominant presence of shorter, more frequent (blue) lightwaves is more likely to be related to a reduction in the experience of pain than is the predominant presence of longer, less frequent (red) lightwaves, or the control condition
2. The longer the duration of exposure to the blue lightwaves, the more likely there will be a reduction in the experience of pain

A convenience sample of 60 female volunteers between the ages of 40 and 60 years who had a medical diagnosis of rheumatoid arthritis and who also reported pain in their left hands at the time of data collection was drawn from persons attending an outpatient rheumatology clinic in the Midwest.

Subjects were randomly assigned to one of six groups. Group 1 had post scores taken in an environment of red lightwaves. Group 2 had post scores taken in an environment of blue lightwaves. Group 3 acted as a control group and had post scores taken in an environment of unfiltered light from the same light source used with the other groups. This source was a standard incandescent household light bulb of 40 watts. Groups 4, 5, and 6 had post-exposure pain scores taken under the same filter conditions as the first three groups, except that these subjects were not able to see the light shining on the study hand during the experimental exposure.

Filters were placed in front of a light bulb held by a metal shade positioned on top of a 3-foot-tall wooden box used to administer the lightwave conditions. This height was used to prevent any influence of heat from the light bulb on subjects' responses. All sides except the top and front of the box were intact. The top was open, but covered with an opaque black cloth while the light was on. The front of the box had a flap-type opening that could be raised and fastened with tape to reveal the light inside, or could be kept shut and sealed when the condition called for the subject to be unable to see the color being shown on the hand. An opening in this wooden flap was covered with black opaque cloth to permit the subject easily to slide the study hand inside the box while blocking the view of the light inside.

The "auditory sensory matching method" was used to measure pain in this study. This method consists of simultaneously comparing the loudness of a tone from a standard clinical audiometer to one's current pain.[17, 21] Subjects were given the instruction, "Turn the dial to find the loudness of the tone that most closely matches the pain in your hand." The intensity of the tone, as measured in decibels, becomes the auditory analogue of the pain. When researchers are attempting to deal with the concept of pain on a unitary basis, a measurement technique must be used that takes into account the emotional as well as the physical aspects of pain.[19, 11, 12] Consequently, this is a most important consideration when using Rogers' model as a conceptual framework in nursing research.

The protocol for the study was as follows: Potential subjects meeting the inclusion criteria were individually approached and given an explanation of the study that met the requirements for informed consent. Demographic information was obtained from the volunteers before they were escorted to a room where the lightwave exposure was administered. The use of the audiometer was explained and demonstrated. Two pre-exposure pain scores were obtained as a reliability check and for covariate use. The subject placed the painful hand in the box containing the lightwaves for 15 minutes. No color names, such as red or blue, were mentioned. Only the term "light" was used by the data collector. Three post scores were obtained at 5-minute intervals during the exposure time. Before the subject was escorted back to the clinic, the investigator answered any questions and changed the filter in preparation for the next subject. The entire participation time averaged 40 minutes.

RESULTS

The overall breakdown of all pre-exposure pain scores showed that subjects randomly placed in the control filter condition had a higher mean score (55.5) than did either the subjects in the red (44.35) or the blue (45.35) filter condition. This difference was not statistically significant by the chi-square test. This result was interpreted as a spurious randomization effect due to the small number of subjects in the study. Differences in the subjects' pre-exposure pain scores based on the presence or absence of a visual barrier were also not significant.

Standard deviations in scores for each group remained similar across all measurements in the study. Those groups that initially showed a higher or lower degree of homogeneity in scores retained that characteristic throughout the study. This consistency was interpreted as evidence supporting the presence of unique differences between people that persist over time and conditions. Even if the overall level of pain in the group changed, no increase in overall uniformity among subjects in the group was obtained.

Hypotheses were tested by two methods. First, a series of multiple analyses of covariance tests were computed by means of the *Statistical Package for the Social Sciences*.[15] The second method used was the multivariate analysis-of-variance technique. This method is a more precise technique of analysis to use with a mixed design study. The pre-exposure pain score was used as a covariate in both tests.

The first hypothesis dealt with the relationship between the predominant presence of blue lightwaves and a reduction in the experience of pain. This hypothesis was supported by results in the predicted direction. The multiple analysis of covariance tests on post scores after a 15-minute exposure produced nonspecific F ratios for the variables of filter (2.417, $p = 0.098$), barrier (0.733, $p = 0.396$), and group (1.839, $p = 0.121$), although the F ratio for the filter variable closely approached the alpha level (0.05) of significance selected for this study. The results of the multivariate analysis of variance test also did not achieve the level for statistical significance, although again the filter variable (F 1.326, p = 0.274) was shown to be more closely related to changes in the dependent measure than was the barrier variable (F 0.499, p = 0.506). No interaction effects were shown to be significant.

Further analysis of the filter variable as related to the first hypothesis was accomplished by examining the mean post-exposure scores of the six groups in the study. When these scores were plotted (Fig. 11–2), it was shown that subjects who were exposed to the blue lightwaves had a greater difference between pre and post scores, and had a consistently progressive decrease in scores as compared to those subjects in the red or control conditions. Differences were also shown between filter conditions when the barrier variable was isolated. The two control groups, one with a barrier and one without, had very different pre scores. However, the curves indicating a response to the lightwaves were very similar. The two blue groups had both similar pre scores and response curves. In contrast, the two red groups had similar pre scores, but differed in response curves. The red group with a barrier had a modest but continuous decline in pain, while the red group without a barrier had an initial decrease in pain followed by a gradual increase, finally reaching a pain level *greater* than the pre score. This response may have been due to an influence of some psychological connotations of the color red as perceived

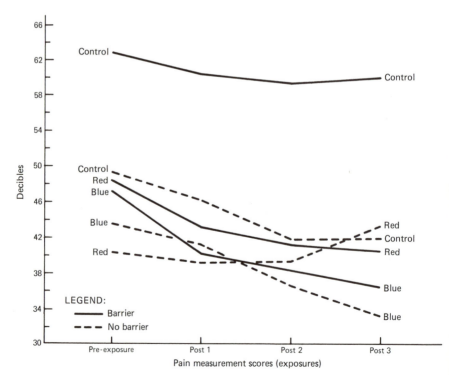

Figure 11–2. Plot of means for each group over pain measurement scores.

by these people. Red is said to have the qualities of excitement, stimulation, energy, and vigor.[3, 4, 14, 19]

The fact that some decrease in pain also occurred in the red and control filter conditions may have been due to a testing or "Hawthorne-like" effect. Or it may have been related to contamination of the lightwave conditions, since entirely monochromatic filters were not used.

The analysis of the effect of the barrier variable on the dependent measure scores showed that the difference between subjects on the post scores was *not* related to the ability to see the light or to know what color was being shown on the study hand during the experiment. This finding supports the postulation that a response to visible lightwaves (colors) is not dependent on the visual process.[13, 20]

The second hypothesis dealt with the variable of time, testing to determine if there was any relationship between the duration of exposure to lightwaves and the experience of pain. This hypothesis was supported by results in the predicted direction and the achievement of an F value of 3.704 ($p = 0.028$) for the time variable in the multivariate analysis-of-variance test. This result suggested that if the lightwave intervention had continued for longer than 15 minutes, a statistically significant result for the filter variable might have been achieved.

DISCUSSION AND RECOMMENDATIONS

Several interesting conclusions related to the development of nursing science can be drawn from the results of this study. These conclusions are relevant to both the applied and the theoretical dimensions of nursing. This demonstrates that a practical nursing intervention can be derived from Rogers' very abstract system. The difficulty in this process lies in the selection of indicators for abstract concepts and the identification or development of appropriate measurement tools for these concepts. Three conclusions relevant to future nursing interventions are suggested by this study. First, blue lightwaves are related to a reduction in the experience of pain in middle-aged women with rheumatoid arthritis. This finding may mean that nurses might assist these clients in using blue lightwaves as a part of their pain-control efforts. Second, the longer the exposure to the blue lightwaves, the more likely there will be a reduction in the experience of pain. This suggests that if lightwaves are used, there should be a plan to use a period of exposure of at least 15 minutes. Third, it is not necessary to see the lightwaves in order to be influenced by them. This suggests that the use of lightwaves while the person is asleep may be effective. Further evidence in support of this apparent effect is found in the phototherapy treatment of infants with hyperbilirubinemia; the infants have their eyes carefully covered while their skin is exposed to lightwaves, resulting in a reduction of the jaundice.[2, 6]

Theory testing is important to nursing science in order to determine the validity of theories derived from conceptual systems. This investigation was based on the conceptual system proposed for nursing by Rogers.[18] The empirical indicators of the human and environmental fields used here were carefully selected to reflect the constructs in that model. Specifically, the focus was on the homeodynamic principle of complementarity contained in the rhythm theory component of the model. The results of this study provide evidence to support that principle.

The relationship between visible lightwaves and the experience of pain should be further explored. It is recommended that the study be replicated to test whether the same findings are obtained. Even better would be a modification of this design that would increase the duration of exposure to the lightwaves from 15 minutes to at least 1/2 hour. This increase in time would allow for increased manifestation of the mutual field process. Previous work has shown that people do not respond instantaneously to change.[7] Another modification would be the use of lightwaves as nearly monochromatic as possible in the experimental conditions in order to eliminate contamination of these conditions with extraneous frequencies.

Other subject populations should be used to test whether the blue lightwave effect differs with variations in age, sex, socioeconomic status, race, and/or geographic location of residence. Adding these variations would serve to extend the generalizability of findings and to identify intervening influences of these variables on the results of this and future studies.

More nursing research efforts are needed that consider both the theoretical and the applied dimensions of the discipline. These will provide linkages between the empirical and abstract levels of knowledge. In this manner the scientific base of knowledge for the profession will develop.

The rhythm theory component of Rogers' model was not conclusively supported by this study. Further work is needed. These recommendations are intended to facilitate that work and to help bring nursing closer to achieving its goal of development of a scientific base for the profession.

REFERENCES

1. Arthritis Foundation: Basic Facts About Arthritis. The Foundation, 1980
2. Behrman RE, Brown AK, Currie MR, et al.: Preliminary report of the committee on phototherapy in the newborn infant. J Pediatr 84:135, 1974
3. Birren F: Light, Color and Environment. New York, Van Nostrand Reinhold, 1969
4. Birren F: Color and Human Response. New York, Van Nostrand Reinhold, 1978
5. Cortes TA: The Investigation of the Relationship Between Lightwaves and Cardiac Rate, doctoral dissertation. New York University, 1975 (unpublished)
6. Cremer RJ, Periigan PW, Richards DH: Influence of light on the hyperbilirubinemia of infants. Lancet 1:1094–1097, 1958
7. Felton G: Effect of time cycle changes on blood pressure and temperature in young women. Nurs Res 19:48–58, 1970
8. Gallert ML: New Light on Therapeutic Energies. London, Clarke & Company, 1966
9. Guilford JP, Smith PC: A system of color preferences. Am J Psychol 62:815–827, 1959
10. Hardy JS: The nature of pain. J Chronic Dis 4:22–51, 1956
11. Jacox AK: Pain: A Source Book for Nurses and Other Health Professionals. Boston, Little, Brown, 1977
12. Johnson JE, Rice VH: Sensory distress components of pain: Implications for the study of clinical pain. Nurs Res 23:203–209, 1974

13. Kruger H: Other Healers, Other Cures. New York, Bobbs-Merrill, 1974
14. Luscher M: The Luscher Color Test. New York, Pocket Books, 1971
15. Nie NH, Hull CH, Jenkins JG, et al. (eds): Statistical Packages for the Social Sciences, 2nd ed. New York, McGraw-Hill, 1970
16. Nourse JC, Welch RB: Emotional attributes of color: A comparison of violet and green. Percept Mot Skills 32:403–406, 1971
17. Peck RE: A precise technique for the measurement of pain. Headache 67:189–194, 1967
18. Rogers ME: An Introduction to the Theoretical Basis for Nursing. Philadelphia, F.A. Davis, 1971
19. Sharpe DT: The Psychology of Color and Design. Totowa, NJ, Littlefield, Adams, 1975
20. Watson K: Supernature. New York, Bantam Books, 1974
21. White JR: Effects of a counterirritant on perceived pain and hand movement in patients with arthritis. Phys Ther 53:956–960, 1973
22. Zborowski M: Cultural components in response to pain. J Soc Issues 8:16–30, 1952

Critique of McDonald's Study

Joyce J. Fitzpatrick

McDonald chose to focus her study on a specific clinical problem, chronic pain associated with rheumatoid arthritis. Basing her hypothesis on the rhythm theory component of Rogers' conceptualization, McDonald argued that the experience of pain was a manifestation of unitary human and environment interaction. She further proposed that alterations in environmental rhythms, i.e., through changes in lightwaves, would be directly related to the human rhythm, i.e., the correlates of pain. The broad theoretical and empirical links proposed by McDonald are reflected in the diagram presented in the chapter.

The major contribution that McDonald made to the research based on Rogers' conceptualization was the extrapolation of the abstract into a specific clinical practice setting. Even more remarkable was McDonald's ability to create links among the most abstract level of nursing science, a classic quasiexperimental research design, and a predominant care problem, pain. Continued examination of the consistencies and inconsistencies among these various levels of abstraction are strongly recommended to advance our scientific pursuits in nursing more rapidly.

This same strength of McDonald's research can also be identified as a weak link. The specific theoretical relationships among concepts of a highly abstract nature have not yet been specified. Although there have been attempts to more fully explicate the rhythm theory component of Rogers' conceptualization, McDonald's work presents just a hint of this. Another related concern regarding this study was the author's discussion of the relevance of these findings to nursing practice. Such suggestions are not warranted yet, as there needs to be more replication and more statistically significant evidence. It appears as if McDonald has extrapolated too much from her data.

In summary, the study represents a good beginning in the effort to extend Rogers' conceptualization to clinical practice. Extension of this research is recommended.

Response
Sharon F. McDonald

Fitzpatrick succinctly identifies the major strengths and limitations of my study. The theoretical relationships among the concepts were assumptions of the study and certainly need to be looked at very closely. I do not disagree with her comments about this conceptualization.

However, I do disagree with her comments about the discussion of the relevance of the study's findings. I think these findings do warrant the suggestions presented. These serve as impetus to further the research that I agree is absolutely necessary. A significant body of evidence is required before one has assurance that the relationship proposed actually exists in any given situation. My personal goal in using Rogers' framework in this study was to demonstrate that it can be extrapolated into clinical nursing practice. That was accomplished.

Critique of McDonald's Study

Violet M. Malinski

McDonald conceptualized her study within rhythm theory derived from Rogers' system and the principle of complementarity (now "integrality"). At the time McDonald was developing her research, little existed in print from Rogers to update her 1970 text, and only Rawnsley's dissertation was available for critique and discussion. The derivation and description of rhythm theory is one area in need of further documentation and refinement.

Color is one manifestation of environmental field patterning and is a wave phenomenon well suited for study within the Science of Unitary Human Beings. McDonald could have linked the hypotheses regarding blue lightwaves more closely to the theoretical framework.

McDonald discussed the difficulties inherent in selecting measures appropriate for the study of unitary human beings from the range of tools currently available, a problem shared by others working within this system. Using a method from psychophysics, auditory sensory matching, she attempted to integrate emotional and physical aspects in her measurement of subjects' perceptions of pain. It is not clear from the discussion how well this method achieves such an integation. Subjects' comprehension of the procedure would be another factor to examine. I wonder if it would be advisable to test the hearing of potential subjects in order to exclude from participation any with hearing problems.

McDonald chose an experimental design. Although contributing to a more rigorous methodology, it poses an interesting conceptual question in light of the acausal, nonlinear nature of the Science of Unitary Human Beings. The researcher choosing such a design needs to be particularly careful with her or his interpretations of the data, as McDonald was. Although she did not randomly sample, McDonald did randomly assign the 60 subjects among the 6 groups.

Results from the use of the barrier conditions support the unitary nature of the interaction with lightwaves as a whole-person phenomenon. Rather than using a box with a light source, a future researcher might examine what happens when the subject is in a room illuminated by lights of the wavelengths (colors) under study. This was done in the Cortes study cited by McDonald, which explored lightwaves and cardiac rates within a different theoretical framework.

McDonald dealt with the time factor, recommending exposures of a minimum of 30 minutes. Given the findings related to the presence–absence of a barrier, it might be productive to modify the lights in a subjects' bedrooms and conduct the study while they are sleeping, as suggested by McDonald.

McDonald's research raises another interesting question. Color is only one manifestation of field patterning. Is the color, reflective of a particular wavelength, the key, or is it the patterning of the human field as it engages in continuous, mutual process with the environmental field—i.e., would all subjects be expected to experience less pain under blue light regardless of their field patterning (higher or lower frequency)? This would be interesting to explore in light of McDonald's finding that the red group with a barrier demonstrated some decline in pain.

McDonald was able to take a very abstract conceptual system at a time when it was less well developed than it is now and demonstrate its potential relevance to practice. Her study raises a number of interesting questions to be explored in future work.

Response

Sharon F. McDonald

I am delighted to concur with Malinski in recognizing that significant work has been accomplished on the rhythm theory component of Rogers' model since my study was done. We shall all benefit from that work. However, more work needs to be done.

Measurement issues continue to be the subject of much debate. The auditory sensory matching technique used in this study was thought to be an appropriate tool, considering the concept of *unitary human being,* because it was not reductionistic in nature. It did not require the subject to think of pain in any of the specific components described in the literature. Rather, it allowed the subject to respond in an individual way, which was assumed to be from an integrated perspective. Giving the subject no specific context for the description of pain allows for an expression of the whole self.

In this study, as well as in any research situation, subjects must understand what they are supposed to do. I think it was important to note that not one of the 60 subjects questioned what to do when given the instruction, "Match the loudness of the tone to the pain in your hand." There was no hesitation or confusion.

Differences in subjects' hearing acuity levels do not influence results unless the period of time for trials is long enough (several months) for a change to occur. This was not the case here. Since subjects stay in the same group for all measurements, their pre and post scores reflect the same acuity level. Therefore, the effect shown in the scores over this brief time can only be related to the independent variable. In this study, it was noted that the control group with a barrier had much higher scores on all measurements and a consistent pattern over time. In the discussion I suggested only that these people possibly had higher pain levels, but in fact, some or all may have had a lesser hearing acuity level, which would account for the difference in mean pain scores for the groups. One could distinguish these two by testing and controlling for hearing acuity level in the study design. This would be important if the question of equal lightwave effect when different intensities of pain are present is being studied.

I selected an experimental design for the study purposefully in order to rigidly control the influence of factors other than the lightwave variable. It was important to do this in order to most clearly demonstrate any lightwave effect. I do not see any great theoretical problem in the use of an experimental design when one is testing relationships, especially when the investigation is in new and controversial areas. I agree with Malinski that the important consideration lies in the interpretation of results. I do not agree that the method of investigation used has a theoretical conflict.

Continuing work based on the findings of this study will deal with less controlled exposures to lightwaves for longer periods of time. I agree with Malinski's suggestion that patterning of the individual's field in relation to the environmental color field pattern is likely a factor in the interaction between them. Future studies may well look at this question.

12

The Relationship of Mystical Experience, Differentiation, and Creativity in College Students

W. Richard Cowling, III

The purpose of this study was an empirical investigation of the principle of helicy proposed in the Science of Unitary Human Beings conceptual system.[24] The variables of mystical experience and differentiation were proposed indices of the diverse pattern characteristic, and creativity was the proposed index of the innovative characteristic. It was hypothesized that these indices would correlate if the characteristics of human field pattern were consonant in the developmental process.

A volunteer sample of 160 college age students (17 to 24 years of age) comprised of both men (31 percent) and women (69 percent) were administered three paper-and-pencil tests: Hood's Mysticism Scale, Factor I; Witkin's Group Embedded Figures Test; and Gough and Heilbrun's Adjective Check List, from which 19 items were extracted to measure creativity as validated by Yonge.

The findings of this study provided mild support for the proposed hypothesis. Mystical experience and creativity were found to be positively related, as were differentiation and creativity. The principle of helicy was supported by this investigation.

BACKGROUND: GENESIS OF PROBLEM FORMULATION

Delineating the research problem was an outgrowth of identifying the variables that seemed phenomenologically congruent with Rogers' conceptualization of unitary human development. Some of the assumptions that had major significance for framing the problem statement included the nonlinear, four-dimensional perspective of space–time, the probabilistic nature of change, and the irreducibility of the human energy field.

The conceptual meanings of the terms *unitary human being, energy field,* and *pattern* were also crucial to understanding what might be observable phenomena. Rogers has defined *energy field* as a fundamental unit and a unifying concept with energy implying its dynamic nature.[26] Pattern is crucial to understanding the energy field because it is the distinguishing characteristic of each field. Continuous pattern change is viewed as diverse and innovative.

Rogers' postulates, known as the Principles of Homeodynamics, further specify the nature and direction of human and environmental change. The principle of helicy was selected as a launching point for testing theory in this study. The principle of helicy specifies "the continuous innovative, probabilistic, increasing diversity of human and environmental field patterns characterized by nonrepeating rhythmicities."[27] A theoretical proposition that is inherent in the principle of helicy is that a positive relationship exists between the field pattern properties of diversity and innovativeness. This theoretical proposition became the central theme of the further progression of problem formulation.

The next major issue that needed to be addressed was the selection of variables that would serve as indicators of the pattern properties. This issue was addressed by examining correlates of unitary human development proposed by Rogers as well as reviewing previous research related to her perspective.[25] The correlates proposed by Rogers suggest movement toward an increasingly diverse field pattern with perceptual features of *timelessness, continuousness, beyond waking, transcendence, visionary,* and *ethereal.*[25] The descriptive language utilized by Rogers implied perceptual features that are also descriptive of various altered states of consciousness. This led me to explore the literature relating to altered states of consciousness. I was struck with the similarity between the vision of reality known as "mystical" and the conceptualization of reality proposed by Rogers as well as that addressed in modern physics.[2, 18, 36, 43]

The four-dimensional nature of mystical experience seemed logically to provide a unique way of experiencing the environment that could be described as diverse. Browning has proposed that mystical experience may be a shift in knowing from three-dimensional space–time to a four-dimensional unitary mode.[1] Ornstein has described mystical experience as beyond the linear mode of consciousness.[22] Further, Ring has conceptualized the near-death experience, encompassing mystical features, as a four-dimensional high frequency domain.[23] Rogers has associated higher frequency with diversity in her conceptual system.[26] She has also noted that "four-dimensional reality is perceived as a synthesis of nonlinear coordinates from which innovative change continuously and evolutionally emerges."[26] The perceptual nature of mysticism has been characterized by Ornstein as a shift from "the analytic, individual, piece-meal approach to knowledge, to a more receptive, holistic mode."[22]

The variable of differentiation was also included in this study because it was logically congruent with the conceptualization of a diverse human field pattern. The ideas of differentiation and negentropy both imply increasing complexity, diversity, and heterogeneity. Rogers has characterized development of human and environmental fields as negentropic.[26] Specifically differentiation is identified by Rogers as a correlate of unitary human development.[25]

The variable of creativity was selected as one indicator of the pattern property of innovation. *Creative, imaginative, innovation, novel, emerging,* and *visionary* are all key descriptors of unitary human development used by Rogers.[24, 26] Human evolution is conceptualized by Rogers as moving from pragmatic to imaginative, suggesting new potentials.[26] Mooney and Land posited somewhat similar views linking creativity to human development as a basic rhythm of life.[17, 19] Sinnot noted "that life itself is the creative process by virtue of its organizing, pattern-forming, questing quality, its most distinctive character."[31] A general proposition of Guilford's theory of creativity is that it is a basic property of all humans, to a greater or lesser degree.[10]

Following identification of the three variables as indicators of unitary human field pattern diversity and innovativeness, the research literature was reviewed for evidence of correlation. The research literature on mystical experience, differentiation, and creativity provided support for a theoretical proposition that diversity and innovativeness are mutual properties of the human field pattern. Since features of mystical experience have been reported in meditation, peak experience, and some forms of drug experience, the literature in these areas was reviewed. Research has shown that such experiences are positively related to creativity.[11, 14, 34, 35, 37] Research reviewed concerning differentiation and creativity suggested a positive relationship between these two variables as well.[20, 33] Thus, the problem statement was formulated to explore the relationship of mystical experience, differentiation, and creativity,

RELATIONSHIP TO THE SCIENCE OF UNITARY HUMAN BEINGS

The specific focal point of this investigation came from the principle of helicy, which specifies that unitary human development is characterized by an increasing complexity and diversity of a continuously innovative, nonrepetitive field wave pattern and organization. Inherent in an open system of complex fields, innovation of field pattern emerges out of diversity of field pattern. Diversity and innovation are mutual pattern characteristics that should correlate, according to the principle of helicy. Consequently, the greater the field pattern diversity, the greater the innovation of the field pattern.

The variables of mystical experience, differentiation, and creativity are human behaviors that are viewed as manifestations of the human–environmental process. The behavior labeled "mystical experience" is phenomenologically described as a transcendent perceptual experience[13] and is conceptualized as a manifestation of human field pattern diversity.[5] Differentiation behavior is a way of perceiving the environment labeled as field–dependent–independent[39] and conceptualized as a manifestation of increasing complexity and diversity and heterogeneity of human field pattern.[5] Creativity is also a perceptual experience of oneself as possessing certain characteristics and is conceptualized as a manifestation of the human field characterized as innovation.[7, 5]

To summarize, the conceptualizations of this investigation based on the Science of Unitary Human Beings are presented:

- *"Human field pattern* is the human mosaic of waves whose dynamic, continuous change is in the direction of diversity and innovation"
- *"Diversity* is an identifiable human field pattern characteristic manifested in mystical experience and differentiation"
- *"Innovation* is an identifiable human field pattern characteristic manifested in creativity"[5]

A central proposition of the investigation was that mystical experience and differentiation comprise a more complete set as an index of diversity of human field pattern than either variable alone. The concept of diversity as having differing forms or qualities is the logical grounding for this proposition. Central to tapping the characteristic of diversity is the number of potential differing forms or qualities within a pattern profile. The range of differing forms or qualities is greater within the combined set of mystical experience and differentiation than in each separately. Multiple manifestations of a diverse human field pattern are documented by the two variables—in particular, the perceptual features of human–environmental unity and separateness. Thus, the main hypothesis of this investigation was that mystical experience and differentiation together would account for a greater portion of variance of creativity than either variable alone.[5]

METHOD

The investigation of the three variables was accomplished by means of a descriptive correlational design. The independent set of variables was comprised of mystical experience and differentiation, and the dependent variable was creativity. Identification of independent and dependent variables was not intended to imply the possibility of a causal connection. The design was chosen to test the statistical relationship of correlation defined as "patterned mutual change."[38] Exploration of patterned mutual change between the variables was one way of testing the principle of helicy as proposed by Rogers.[24, 26]

The Mysticism Scale, Factor I (M Scale I) developed by Hood was chosen as a measure of mystical experience.[12] Factor II items were not included because they dealt with the concept of religious interpretation.

The scale encompasses eight categories and consists of two negatively expressed items and two positively expressed items for each category. The eight categories are labeled "qualities" and are described here. *Ego Quality* refers to the experience of a loss of sense of self, often accompanied by an absorption into something greater. *Unifying Quality* refers to an experience of a unification of the multiplicity of objects of perception. *Inner Subjective Quality* refers to the perception of living characteristics in all objects. *Temporal–Spatial Quality* refers to an experience in which space and time are modified, sometimes to the extreme of "timelessness" or "spacelessness." *Noetic Quality* refers to the experience as a source of valid knowledge with emphasis on a nonrational, intuitive, insightful experience, yet not merely subjective. *Ineffability Quality* refers to the impossibility of expressing the experience in conventional language. *Positive Affect Quality* is self-explanatory. *Religious Quality* refers to an experience of intrinsic sacredness felt as a mystery, awe, and reverence that may be expressed independently of traditional religious language.[12]

Hood has presented some evidence of construct validity by demonstrating significant correlation ($r = 0.47$, $p < 0.01$, $N = 52$) with the Religious Experience Episodes Measure and with a scale by Taft that shares some conceptual overlap ($r = -0.75$, $p < 0.01$, $N = 83$).[12] The negative correlation in the later study is due to the opposite directions of scoring. Alpha reliability coefficient for the M Scale I in the Cowling study was 0.82.[5]

The Group Embedded Figures Test (GEFT), developed by Witkin, Oltman, Raskin, and Karp, was utilized as the measure of differentiation.[41] The test requires the subject to locate a simple structure in a complex field.

The test was standardized on a group of 168 male and 169 female undergraduate students. For both males and females, internal consistency reliability coefficients were found to be 0.82.[41] In the Cowling investigation, an Alpha reliability coefficient of 0.89 was found.[5]

The measure of creativity chosen was the creativity scale of the Adjective Check List (Cr Scale ACL).[9, 42] Yonge extracted a 19-item scale for creativity from the ACL based on items that discriminated between groups and controls in earlier studies.[6, 32, 42] On a sample of 80 undergraduates, a Kuder-Richardson 21 reliability of 0.83 was reported for the following 19-adjective scale: artistic, assertive, clever, complicated, cynical, idealistic, imaginative, impulsive, ingenious, insightful, intelligent, inventive, original, quick, reflective, resourceful, sharp-witted, spontaneous, and unconventional.[42] For the Cowling investigation, the Alpha reliability coefficient for the Cr Scale ACL was 0.85.[5]

The sample included undergraduates enrolled in introductory psychology classes in a community college located in a southeastern city of approximately 100,000 population. The sample size was 160, yielding a power greater than 0.98 to detect a medium effect ($f_2 = 0.15$) at the 0.05 level in a three-variable multiple regression analysis.[3] The sample size is also consistent with the recommendation of at least 30 subjects for each predicator variable to minimize shrinkage of R^2.[16]

The majority of the subjects were women (69 percent) and were in the age range of 18 to 19 years (61 percent). While 38 percent of the subjects were aged 21 to 24, only 1 percent were 17 years of age. A wide array of college majors was unevenly represented by the sample. Participation and nonparticipation in religious activities was approximately balanced for the sample, with Protestant denominational affiliations predominantly represented. Current use of medications (depressants, stimulants, or hallucinogens) was reported by 8 percent of the sample.

Information about meditation practices was also solicited by the researcher because of the linkage of meditation with mystical experience and creativity in the literature.[18, 22] While it appeared that 8 percent ($N = 12$) of the subjects practiced some form of meditation, inconsistency in individual responses to the series of questions yielded ambiguous findings overall. The implication of problematic wording was suggested by the many questions raised by subjects during the completion of this area of the form.

All subjects were tested in a classroom setting in groups ranging in size from 12 to 41 subjects. Testing was done by the investigator or a trained assistant in compliance to a preformulated testing procedure. The investigator or a trained assistant was introduced to the group by the class instructor or professor. The voluntary nature of the testing was emphasized after briefly describing the purpose of the study. Folders were distributed containing an explanation and consent form, a coded demographic information form, and coded tests of the three variables.

RESULTS

The mean score for the M Scale I, GEFT, and Cr Scale ACL for the sample were generally consistent with published norms for the three tests.[12, 41, 42] Skewness was near zero for the M Scale I and GEFT and slightly positive for the Cr Scale ACL. Correlation coefficients among the variables are presented in Table 12–1.

A significant (0.01) positive linear relationship between mystical experience and creativity as well as a significant (0.05) positive linear relationship between differentiation and creativity as measured by the instrumentation of the study was found, based on computation of the t statistic. The negative relationship between mystical experience and differentiation was nonsignificant. Thus, while there were significant positive linear relationships between the individual independent variables and the dependent variables, there were no significant linear relationships between the two independent variables.

Results of the multiple regression analysis showed that approximately 14.5 percent ($R^2 = 0.14509$, $p < 0.001$, $F = 13.32$, $df = 2,157$) of the total variance in creativity was accounted for by the linear combination of mystical experience and differentiation. Beta weights for the M Scale I and GEFT were 0.34304 and 0.18445 consecutively.

The hypothesis was tested by computation of an F ratio for significance in the difference between the coefficient of determination (r) for each independent variable with the dependent variable and the coefficient of determination for the multiple regression (R^2). Computation of the F statistic for the coefficient of determination for mystical experience and creativity yielded $F = 6.80$ ($df = 1,157$), which is significant at the 0.05 level. The F statistic computed for the coefficient of determination for differentiation and creativity was $F = 2.347$ ($df = 1,157$), which is significant at the 0.01 level. Thus, support was found for the hypothesis that mystical experience and differentiation together (linear combination) account for a greater portion of variance of creativity than either variable alone.

TABLE 12–1. CORRELATION COEFFICIENTS: MYSTICISM SCALE (FACTOR I), GROUP EMBEDDED FIGURES TEST, AND CREATIVITY SCALE OF ADJECTIVE CHECK LIST ($N = 160$)

	GEFT	Cr Scale ACL
M scale I	−0.052	0.333*
GEFT	————	0.167†

*$p < 0.01$.
†$p < 0.05$.

DISCUSSION AND RECOMMENDATIONS

The findings of the study were that: (1) mystical experience and creativity together accounted for a greater portion of variance of creativity than either variable alone; (2) mystical experience and differentiation together accounted for a relatively small portion (14.5 percent) of the variance of creativity; (3) a greater portion of variance in creativity was accounted for by mystical experience (11 percent) than by differentiation (3 percent); (4) mystical experience and creativity were positively related; (5) differentiation and creativity were positively related; (6) mystical experience and differentiation were orthogonal; and (7) mystical experience and differentiation did not interact to influence creativity. All these findings are interpreted in the context of the parameters of the present study, including sample characteristics and measure of variables.

The main finding of the study represents mild support for the hypothesis of the study and consequently contributes theoretical support for Rogers' principle of helicy, which postulates unitary human development characterized by increasingly diverse and innovative field patterning.[41] It was hypothesized that indices of these pattern characteristics would correlate. Evidence of patterned mutual change between the variables was represented by the correlational findings through hypothesis testing.[38] Thus, the concept of mutuality of field pattern characteristics as postulated in the principle of helicy is supported by the correlational findings.

Tentative support for the conceptualization of a diverse human field pattern as proposed by the investigator is also given by the main finding. It was suggested that central to measuring the characteristic of diversity is the number of potential differing forms or qualities within a pattern profile. The idea that the two independent variables document a wider range of manifestations of the diverse human field pattern was supported because the correlation to the proposed index of innovative field pattern was higher for the linear combination of mystical experience and differentiation than for each variable separately.

The second finding, the low portion of variance in creativity accounted for by mystical experience and differentiation, may indicate that while these two variables represent a higher degree of diversity than either separately, they do not adequately represent the full spectrum of human qualities of a diverse field pattern. While mystical experience and differentiation appear to document some unique manifestations of a diverse human field pattern, the addition of other variables may be necessary to encompass the full attributes of the pattern profile. Rogers has suggested that events labeled "paranormal" as well as rhythmical correlates of change such as sleep–wake patterns are worth considering as manifestations of the human field pattern. Others have proposed exploring experiential states manifest in dreams, fantasy, meditation, serious illness, peak experiences, movement, music, solitude, and intellectual struggle.[8, 30]

The foregoing explanation was based upon the assumption that creativity is an adequate index of the innovative pattern profile. Conversely, if one assumes that the design allows for the accurate representation of diversity, the low multiple correlation coefficient may be attributed to the inadequacy of creativity as an index of the innovative pattern profile.

The low correlation appears to support the suggestion by Ference that "if the principle of helicy is operational, the indices of human development may be constant but the relative direction and degree may vary with other conditions."[8] While the indices of a diverse and innovative field pattern were constant, there was a high degree of variance among the subjects. In other words, the magnitude of correlation in the sample indicates that there was a large variety of pattern profiles representing varying degrees of diversity and innovativeness. Again, such an interpretation is consistent with the distinguishing feature of diversity as possessing differing forms or qualities.

The third finding was that the greater portion of variance in creativity was accounted for by mystical experience (11 percent) rather than by differentiation (3 percent). Earlier research has led investigators to assume that the GEFT measures a broad dimension of human development with diverse manifestations.[40] Also, research has suggested a relative strong positive relationship between differentiation and creativity[10, 21, 33] and a weaker relationship between mystical experience and creativity.[4, 7, 34, 35] The third finding suggests that mystical experience may represent a broader dimension of unitary development than differentiation as measured in this study.

One possible explanation is that mystical experience may encompass qualities more closely associated with the innovative field pattern characteristic of unitary human development. Although the principle of resonancy was not the focus of the investigation, it may help explain the difference in correlations for mystical experience and differentiation with creativity.[26] Resonancy postulates that human fields manifest change in the direction of higher wave frequency patterns. Further, Rogers has noted that higher wave frequencies are characterized by diversity and innovative field pattern.[25, 26] It is possible that mystical experiences may be reflective of relatively higher frequency wave patterns than differentiation qualities. Such an explanation has theoretical support from Ring, who proposed that the core experience of near-death is a type of mystical experience in which one becomes sensitive to a higher frequency domain.[23]

The fourth and fifth findings—that positive relationships exist between mystical experience and creativity, and between differentiation and creativity—will be discussed simultaneously. A positive relationship demonstrates that the variables covary in the same direction. The implication of these findings for the principle of helicy is that there is congruent directionality of the diverse and innovative field pattern properties demonstrated in this sample by covariance of indices of these pattern properties.

In light of the sixth finding, mystical experience and differentiation appear to be unique individual dimensions of unitary human development. The fact that there was no significant linear relationship between mystical experience and differentiation indicates that they may tap different parameters of the field pattern and organization. Again, this finding is congruent with the researcher's logic that two differing variables comprise greater diversity than a single variable. The range of differing qualities represented by two variables that have an independent relationship is potentially greater than if they are not independent.

The seventh finding—that mystical experience and differentiation did not interact to influence creativity—also has implications for Rogers' conceptual system. It gives further support for the idea that mystical experience and differentiation may be separate dimensions of field pattern and organization because it demonstrates the each variable accounts for variance in creativity in its own way. The joint effects of two noninteracting variables are described as additive.[15]

Recommendations are provided for the continued development and explication of the Science of Unitary Human Beings. Further examination of the measures employed in this study for compatibility with Rogers' construct is crucial to improve the quality of future research. Specifically, studies exploring the relationship of the M Scale I to measures that have face-validity as derived from Rogers' framework, such as the human field motion scale, might provide evidence of construct validity.[8] In addition, test developments aimed at the field pattern properties of diversity and innovation are needed. Indices of human field pattern that have potential value for further exploration include sleep–wake patterns, dream states, extrasensory perception, clairvoyance, near-death phenomena, and paranormal events.

REFERENCES

1. Browning R: Psychotherapeutic Change East and West: Buddhist Psychological Paradigm of Change with Reference to Psychoanalysis, doctoral dissertation. California School of Professional Psychology, 1978 (Dissertation Abstracts International 39:6110B, 1979)
2. Capra F: The Tao of Physics. Berkley, Shambala, 1975
3. Cohen J: Statistical Power Analysis for the Behavioral Sciences. New York, Academic Press, 1977
4. Cowger EL: The Effect of Meditation (Zazen) upon Selected Dimensions of Personal Development, doctoral dissertation. University of Georgia, 1973 (Dissertation Abstracts International 34:4734A, 1974)
5. Cowling R: The Relationship of Mystical Experience, Differentiation, and Creativity in College Students: An Empirical Investigation of the Principle of Helicy in Rogers'

Science of Unitary Human Beings. doctoral dissertation. New York University, 1983 (University Microfilms Publication No: 84-06, 283)

6. Domino G: Identification of Potentially Creative Persons from the Adjective Check List. J Consult Clin Psychol 35:48–51, 1970
7. Domino G: Transcendental Meditation and Creativity: An Empirical Investigation. J Appl Psychol 66:358–362, 1977
8. Ference H: The Relationship of Time Experience, Creativity Traits, Differentiation, and Human Field Motion: An Empirical Investigation of Rogers' Correlates of Synergistic Human Development, doctoral dissertation. New York University, 1979 (University Microfilms Publication No: 80-10, 281)
9. Gough HG, Heilburn AB: The Adjective Checklist Manual. Palo Alto, Consulting Psychologists Press, 1965
10. Guilford JP: A psychometric approach to creativity. In Bloomberg M (ed): Creativity: Theory and Research. New Haven, Conn, College & University Press, 1973
11. Harman WW, McKim RH, Mogar RE, et al.: Psychedelic agents in creative problem solving. In Tart CT (ed): Altered States of Consciousness. New York, Wiley, 1969
12. Hood RW Jr: The construction and preliminary validation of a measure of reported mystical experience. J Sci Study Religion 14:29–41, 1975
13. Hood RW Jr: Eliciting mystical states of consciousness with semistructured nature experiences. J Sci Study Religion 16:155–163, 1977
14. Hood RW Jr, Hall JR, Watson PJ, et al.: Personality correlates of the report of mystical experience. Psychol Rep 44:804–806, 1979
15. Keppel G: Design and Analysis: A Researcher's Handbook. Englewood Cliffs, NJ, Prentice-Hall, 1973
16. Kerlinger FN, Pedhazur EJ: Multiple Regression in Behavioral Research. New York, Holt, Rinehart, & Winston, 1973
17. Land DTL: Grow or Die: The Unifying Principle of Transformation. New York, Delta, 1973
18. LeShan L: The Medium, the Mystic, and the Physicist. New York, Ballantine, 1966
19. Mooney RL: A conceptual model for integrating four approaches to the identification of creative talent. In Taylor CW, Barron F (eds): Scientific Creativity: Its Recognition and Development. New York, Wiley, 1963
20. Morris TL, Bergum BO: A note on the relationship between field-independence and creativity. Percep Mot Skills 46:1114, 1978
21. Noppe LD, Gallagher JM: A cognitive style approach to creative thought. J Pers Assess 41:85–90, 1977
22. Ornstein RE: The Psychology of Consciousness. New York, Penguin Books, 1972
23. Ring K: Life and Death: A Scientific Investigation of the Near-Death Experience. New York, Coward, McCann, & Geoghegan, 1980
24. Rogers ME: An Introduction to the Theoretical Basis of Nursing. Philadelphia, F. A. Davis, 1970
25. Rogers ME: Postulated Correlates of Unitary Human Development. New York University, 1979 (unpublished)
26. Rogers ME: Nursing: A Science of Unitary Man. In Riehl JP, Roy C (eds): Conceptual Models for Nursing Practice, 2nd ed. New York, Appleton-Century-Crofts, 1980
27. Rogers ME: Nursing Science: A Science of Unitary Man: Glossary. New York University, 1982 (unpublished)
28. Sandford DE: Inspiration in the Creative Process and Meditation, doctoral dissertation. The Johns Hopkins University, 1975 (Dissertation Abstracts International, 39:2481B, 1978)

29. Shecter HE: A Psychological Investigation into the Source of the Effect of the Transcendental Meditation Technique, doctoral dissertation. York University, Canada, 1977 (Dissertation Abstracts International, 38:3372B–337B, 1978)

30. Shetler EAB: Nursing conceptual frameworks as bases for research. Paper presented at the meeting of Upsilon Chapter, Sigma Theta Tau, New York University, November 1980

31. Sinnot E: The creativeness of life. In Anderson HH (ed): Creativity and Its Cultivation. New York, Harper & Row, Pub, 1959

32. Smith JM, Schaefer CE: Development of a creativity scale for the adjective check list. Psychol Rep 25:87–92, 1969

33. Spotts JV, Mackler B: Relationships of field dependent and field independent cognitive styles to creative test performance. Percep Mot Skills 24:239–168, 1967

34. Taft R: Peak experiences and ego permissiveness. Acta Psychol 29:35–64, 1969

35. Taft R: The Measurement of the Dimensions of Ego Permissiveness. Pers: Internat J 1:163–184, 1970

36. Talbot M: Mysticism and the New Physics. New York, Bantam Books, 1980

37. Travis F: The transcendental meditation technique and creativity: A longitudinal study of Cornell University undergraduates. J Creative Behav 13:169–180, 1979

38. Walizer MH, Weiner PL: Research Methods and Analysis: Searching for Relationships. New York, Harper & Row, 1979

39. Witkin HA, Dyke RB, Faterson HF, et al.: Psychological Differentiation. New York, Wiley, 1962

40. Witkin HA, Goodenough DR, Oltman PK: Psychological Differentiation: Current Status. Research Bulletin No. 77–17. Princeton, NJ, Educational Testing Services, 1977

41. Witkin HA, Oltman PK, Raskin E, et al.: Manual for the Embedded Figures Tests. Palo Alto, Consulting Psychologists Press, 1971

42. Younge CD: Time experiences, self-actualizing values, and creativity. J Pers Assess 39:601–606, 1975

43. Zukav G: The Dancing Wu Li Masters: An Overview of the New Physics. New York, Morrow, 1979

Critique of Cowling's Study

Joyce J. Fitzpatrick

Cowling has focused on Rogers' principle of helicy in explicating the rationale for this study. Mystical experience and differentiation were conceptually linked to diversity, and creativity was linked to innovation. Cowling clearly described the process for deriving the indicators. This description would have been aided by more detail about the logical deduction process. For example, Cowling suggested that theory development was a focal point in this process, but has not outlined here either the specific theory development process or the theoretical formulations that were derived. The reader would have benefited also from the provision of supporting data from other research. While Cowling proposed a similarity in Rogers' conceptualization and that of mysticism, one cannot be certain what this similarity was. Further, no research literature is critiqued in relation to these variables.

One of the major strengths of the Cowling study was the explicit description of the relationship of this research to Rogers' conceptual model. Rogers' assumptions, principle of helicy, and conceptual descriptions of patterns were fully explicated. Such a description should be of particular benefit to the novice student of Rogers. Statements were clear and direct and seemed to leave little question about conceptual fit.

Cowling's research also was built on the work of others; he obviously benefited from careful study of both Rogers' conceptual system and the work of his predecessors. What was less clear here was the broader context of nursing in which this research was cast. Cowling did not attempt to relate this research to the nursing practice dimension. It did not appear as if this would be difficult. One wonders why there was a lack of attention to this concern.

In this research report, Cowling discussed, in moderate detail, some of the psychometric qualities of the instruments used. He appeared not to have some of the measurement problems of some other investigators. Concern could be raised about inclusion of only self-perception self-report measures. Inclusion of additional measures presents a challenge for future research. Cowling also noted some possible problem in interpretation of additional questions of meditation; apparently such questions had various meanings attached. Cowling appropriately raised other questions regarding instrumentation in relation to the concepts and variables for this study.

Generally, Cowling's conclusions are supported by the data. Only occasionally does he go beyond the data; even then the discussion was framed as speculation. Cowling further proposed, however, that we concern ourselves with methods and measures. Recommendations for future research were realistic. In addition, they may hold great potential to clarify this area of interest.

Response

W. Richard Cowling, III

Fitzpatrick's critique has highlighted some of the strengths and weaknesses of the report of the investigation, as well as the investigation itself. The critique provides an opportunity to explicate the particularly unexplicit features of the investigation as reported.

The focal point of theory development was to derive a testable theorem (in the form of the hypothesis) from the principle of helicy, which is a generalization concerning the nature of unitary human development. The identification of variables that were proposed as indices of diversity and innovativeness enabled the researcher to test a theory of field pattern diversity that may have been more simply stated as: The experiential features of mystical experience and differentiation represent a fuller spectrum of diversity than either variable alone. Consequently, a higher correlation with the mutual field pattern characteristic of innovativeness.

The lack of inclusion of supporting evidence from previous research in the report is a function of both the presentation format requirement and space limitations. Fitzpatrick's concern is justified. The researcher provided a comprehensive review of supporting research in the study text.

The major conceptual connection between Rogers and mystical experience is the striking similarity in language used by Rogers to describe correlates of unitary development and the phenomenological description of reality by mystical "experiencers." Examples of the congruent descriptors are: continuous, transcendent, ethereal, timeless, and beyond waking.

The relationship of the study to the nursing practice dimension can be described in several areas. The phenomenological features of mystical experience are also evidenced in states labeled as "psychological disorder," near-death experiences, dreaming, peak experiences, drug-related states, flow experiences associated with exercise, and meditation. There is also mounting evidence that these phenomenological experiences comprise a part of ordinary life experience on a daily basis. The relationship of these experiences to health have only been superficially addressed. An understanding of mystical experiences seems relevant to addressing the full potential of humans that we serve. Rogers' conceptual framework is only one particular explanatory context for the mystical experience.

The inclusion of only self-report, self-perception measures was purposive in this particular investigation and arose from the researcher's epistemological stance based on Rogers' perspective of human nature. Self-perception, self-report measures of variables was a favored methodology in this research study because the aim was to tap the direct experiencing features of unitary development. Fitzpatrick's comments suggest a need for greater clarity in reporting, which emphasizes the logic of methodological choices.

13

The Relationship of Creativity, Actualization, and Empathy in Unitary Human Development

Martha Raile Alligood

The purpose of this study was to describe the relationships of creativity and actualization with empathy. These three variables were proposed as manifestations of helicy, Rogers' principle of unitary human development. Helicy states that development is continuously innovative and characterized by diversity of field pattern in relation to the continuous, mutual process of human and environmental fields.[23]

This beginning descriptive study proposed to test Rogers' principle of helicy by measuring individuals for manifestations of helicy. A volunteer sample of 236 persons participated by completing paper-pencil tests that were measures of innovativeness manifest as creativity, increasing diversity manifest as actualization, and the human–environment process manifest as empathy.

The findings support the hypotheses. Creativity and actualization are each positively correlated with empathy. Further, the two combined account for more variance than either did separately. This further supports the principle of helicy, because each variable (manifestation) represents a distinct characteristic of helical development as proposed in the principle. Therefore, the lack of homeoscedasticity in their relationships with empathy accounts for more variance in empathy, as well as being supportive of the principle. Creativity, actualization, and empathy are suggested as field pattern manifestations of helicy in developing human beings.

BACKGROUND: GENESIS OF PROBLEM FORMULATION

Rogers' system provides the basis for a Science of Unitary Human Beings. The concepts of energy field, open systems, pattern, and four-dimensionality provide a framework for investigations of unitary human development. Studies within the conceptual system yield knowledge to direct and support nursing.

The principle of helicy put forward by Rogers provides the rationale for the identification of the manifestations and their proposed relationships.[23] This study was designed to describe the relationships of creativity and actualization with empathy. These three variables were proposed as manifestations of human field pattern in unitary human development. The nature of human beings and their unitary development is of central concern to nursing. Therefore, human beings are the phenomenon of study for nursing science.

Rogers' Science of Unitary Human Beings was the conceptual framework for this study. Helicy describes development as continuously innovative and characterized by diversity of field pattern in relation to the continuous mutual process between the human and environmental field.[23] Using Rogers' principle of helicy, I proposed the following as a descriptive study for the measurement of helicy, through manifestations, in human development.

Since helicy states the nature and direction of development is (1) innovative, (2) increasingly diverse, and (3) emerging out of the continuous mutual process of human beings and environment, these three characteristics were identified as manifestations to test for the presence of the principle of helicy in developing individuals.

Innovative field pattern was proposed to manifest human creativity in individual expressions of the tendency toward variety. The increasing diversity of field pattern was proposed to manifest human actualization as individual emergence of human potential. The continuous, mutual process of the human and environmental fields was proposed to manifest empathy in individuals as feeling attributes.

Therefore, creativity, actualization, and empathy were proposed as manifestations of unitary human development. The principle of helicy not only suggests the presence of these three manifestations in developing humans, but also suggests a positive relationship of creativity and actualization with empathy.

This study proposed to test helicy by testing for the presence of the manifestations in individuals and predicting their relationships based on Rogers' Science of Unitary Human Beings and particularly the principle of helicy. The principle was used for the identification of manifestations one could expect to be present. Further, the proposed relationships of the three manifestations were derived from the principle of helicy as it sets forth its characteristics. From the problem statement, "What is the relationship among creativity, actualization, and empathy?" the following hypotheses were derived:[20]

1. There is a positive correlation between creativity and empathy
2. There is a positive correlation between actualization and empathy
3. Creativity and actualization, combined, will account for more of the variance in empathy than either one will separately

Helicy suggests that innovativeness and increasing diversity emerge in relation to the human and environmental process. Therefore, one could theorize that each of these manifestations would be positively correlated with empathy. Further, as manifestations of different characteristics of helicy, one could theorize that creativity and actualization would combine to account for more variance than either of the manifestations accounted for individually. Therefore, this study proposed to test for the presence of identified manifestations of helicy that represented separate characteristics and shared little covariance. Also, it proposed to test for the direction of development that helicy specified to be positive.

Rogers' conceptual system provided the rationale for this study. However, because nursing science is in the beginning stage of development, the related literature was searched and studied with regard to each variable and the relationships among the variables as reported in the literature. From the related literature, Maslow[12–14] and Carl Rogers[22] supported the testing of the relationship between creativity and empathy and between actualization and empathy. Taylor, Crutchfield, and Vargiu reported a relationship between the former.[1, 25, 27] Lash, Fischer, and Rodriguez suggested a relationship between the latter.[5, 11, 21] The relationship between creativity and actualization was also tested in the present study, since the literature suggested the need for further exploration. However, the independent variables were truly independent, as no relationship was found. No study was found that tested the relationships proposed among the three variables in this study.

RELATIONSHIP TO THE SCIENCE OF UNITARY HUMAN BEINGS

Rogers discussed unitary human development in principles that are postulated to describe the nature and direction of human development. Rogers' definition of helicy was utilized for the identification of manifestations to be measured. Further, the proposed relationships among the three manifestations derived from helicy as it sets forth characteristics. These characteristics suggested human behaviors that could be theorized to manifest helicy in unitary human development.

Helicy suggests that innovativeness and increasing diversity emerge in relation to the continuous, mutual human–environment process. Creativity is a manifestation of innovative human field pattern. Rogers has stated, "Change is always innovative."[23] Creativity is, therefore, inherent in the conceptual system and in helicy. Since behavior manifests the unitary human field, it follows that there should be a manifestation of innovativeness in human development as postulated in helicy. It is proposed that creativity, characterized by a tendency toward variety, is a manifestation of innovative human field pattern.

Actualization is a manifestation of increasing diversity of human field pattern. Rogers says, "There are multiple evidences of man's developmental potentials in process of actualization."[23] If this is true of development in general, there must also be a unitary manifestation of the emerging developmental potentials. Actualization is proposed as a unitary manifestation of the increasing diversity of field pattern characterized by evolving human potentialities.

The manifestation of the characteristics of creativity as innovative human field pattern and actualization as increasing diversity of human field pattern is associated with another human field pattern of helicy, which is manifest as *empathy*. Empathy is a human field pattern manifestation emerging from the mutual human being–environment process. Helicy specifies the human being–environment process to be continuous and mutual. Human beings and environment are integral and change together. Empathy is proposed as a human field pattern manifestation characterized by feeling attributes. Rogers identifies feelings as behavior of the unitary human field.[23] Therefore, empathy is proposed as a unitary evidence of the feelings characteristic of the mutual human being–environment process.

METHOD

To test the relationships among the variables, three paper-pencil tests were administered. Each of the three tests provided a single score for each participant on each variable. Correlations of the scores were used to test the relationships among the variables in a sample of 236 women and men between 18 and 60 years of age. Table 13–1 shows the demographic data that provides a description of the sample. The Personal Orientation Inventory (POI) was used as the measure of actualization.[24] The test is designed to measure evolving potential through forced-choice answers to 150 dichotomous questions. Evolving potential is a characteristic of in-

TABLE 13–1. A DESCRIPTION OF THE SAMPLE FROM THE DEMOGRAPHIC INFORMATION FORM WITH THE _N_ AND THE PERCENTAGES FOR THE GROUPS OF EACH CATEGORY (_N_ = 236)

Categories	N	%
Age		
18–30	44	19
31–40	85	36
41–50	74	31
51–60	33	14
Sex		
Female	155	66
Male	81	34
Country of Birth		
United States	234	99
Other	2	1
Country of Residence		
United States	232	98
Other	4	2
State of Residence		
Ohio	157	66
Indiana	30	13
Tennessee	12	5
Florida	6	3
Pennsylvania	5	2
Missouri	5	2
Illinois	5	2
Kentucky	5	2
Michigan	2	1
Texas	1	0.4

Categories	N	%
Alabama	2	1
Nebraska	1	0.4
Other than United States	4	2
No response	1	0.4
Description of Residence		
Rural	81	34
Town	53	23
City	54	23
Suburban	38	16
Metropolitan	10	4
Occupation		
Professional, technical, and managerial	87	37
Clerical and sales	35	15
Service	72	30
Agriculture, forestry	4	2
Processing	2	1
Machine trade	3	1
Benchwork	8	3
Structural work	4	2
Miscellaneous	17	7
No response	4	2
Education		
Grade school	4	2
High school	60	25
Vocational	14	6
Some college	59	25
Associate degree	14	6
Bachelors degree	46	20
Masters degree	27	11
Doctorate	8	3
Other	4	2

creased diversity in unitary human development, which is manifest as actualization. The 127 item I-scale for the POI was used as an overall single measure of actualization. Validity and reliability are well established.[2, 3]

The Similes Preference Inventory was used as the measure of creativity.[19] The test is designed to measure the tendency toward variety through the choice of endings for 54 similes. The tendency toward variety is a characteristic of the innovativeness of human development.

The Hogan scale was used to measure empathy.[7] The test is designed to measure the feeling attributes of empathy through 39 true-and-false questions. The feeling attributes of empathy are a characteristic of the mutual human–environment process.

The hypotheses of this study proposed the relationships of the three variables of creativity, actualization, and empathy. Creativity, actualization, and empathy were proposed as behaviors that emerge as manifestations of the field pattern of human beings and environment.

Given the relationships of the three characteristics within the principle of helicy, it followed that each independent variable should relate positively with empathy, the dependent variable. Further, it was proposed that the independent variables, combined, would account for more of the variance in empathy than either one did separately.

Data were collected from volunteers at a large Christian convention and from Christian churches in the Midwest. The volunteers were told that participation would take approximately 1 hour while they completed a demographic information form and three paper-pencil tests. The following explanation of the purpose of the study was given: "Because the focus of nursing is unitary man, nurses need basic knowledge about human development. This study is designed to describe the relationship among three behaviors that are proposed as evidences of human development. The information that will come from the results of the study should contribute to the knowledge base for nursing."

A consent form insuring willingness to participate and informing participants of their right to withdraw at any time was completed by the volunteers before the tests were taken. Confidentiality of the participants was maintained by assigning an identification number to each answer sheet and demographic information form prior to testing. Participants were informed verbally that the identification number was being used to assure the anonymity of their answers. On the consent form participants were given a choice of whether to have a summary of the results of the study sent to them. If they chose yes, they were asked to provide their names and addresses. Participants were asked to complete the tests in the order they appeared in their folders. The three tests were ordered in one of the six possible orders to rule out test effects.

RESULTS

Data were analyzed as follows: The Similes Preference Inventory, the Hogan Scale, and the Personal Orientation Inventory were scored, and each test yielded a single score for each individual.

A Pearson Correlation subprogram of Bivariate Correlation Analysis and a Regressions subprogram of Multiple Regression Analysis from the *Statistical Package for the Social Sciences,* Version H, Release 9, were used to test the hypotheses.[18] Hypotheses, correlation coefficients, and percentage of covariance are shown in Table 13–2. For hypotheses 1 and 2, data were analyzed by computing the Pearson product–moment correlation coefficients to test the relationship of creativity to empathy and the relationship of actualization to empathy. For hypothesis 3, multiple regression was used to test if the magnitude of the multiple R was greater than the Pearson r when creativity and actualization, combined, were related to empathy. Significance of the correlation was tested by computing the F test with acceptance set at the 0.05 level.

The positive relationship of creativity with empathy as hypothesized is illustrated with the coefficient of 0.269. Whereas the magnitude of this Pearson prod-

TABLE 13–2. HYPOTHESES, CORRELATION COEFFICIENTS, AND PERCENTAGE OF COVARIANCE ($N = 236$)

Hypothesis	Correlation	% of Covariance
1	0.269*	7
2	0.391*	15
3	0.461*	21

*$p < 0.001$.

uct–moment correlation coefficient is in the low range, it may be regarded as indicating a low degree of correlation and does demonstrate the presence of a relationship. This finding supports the theoretical relationship between innovativeness and the human–environment process that was postulated in the principle of helicy. The related literature had also suggested the possibility of a relationship between creativity and empathy.[23, 25]

The positive relationship of actualization with empathy as hypothesized is illustrated with a coefficient of 0.391. Whereas the magnitude of this Pearson product–moment correlation coefficient is in the moderate range, it may be regarded as indicating a moderate degree of correlation and does demonstrate the presence of a relationship. This finding supports the theoretical relationship between increasing diversity and the human–environment process that was postulated by helicy. The finding of relationship in the present study also supports the relationship reported in the related literature.[5, 11]

The first two hypotheses were supported and, although the correlation coefficients are low to moderate, they were highly significant ($p < 0.001$), which demonstrates their stability. Further, the lack of relationship between the two independent variables contributes to the value of the findings, since each variable is accounting for little variance in empathy accounted for by the other variable.

The multiple R for the relationship of creativity and actualization combined with empathy was 0.461. The meaning of the multiple correlation comes from the percentage of variance explained. Whereas the magnitude of the multiple R accounted for only 21 percent of the variance in empathy, the $F (2,233) = 31.41$ indicated stability. Further, the F ratio used to test the significance of the difference between the R^2 for the first step and the R^2 for the second step in the multiple regression was $F (1,234) = 17.65$ and was significant beyond the 0.01 level. The findings of relationship of creativity and actualization to empathy support the relationship of innovativeness and increasing diversity to the human–environment process as postulated by helicy. These findings of relationship also support the ideas of Land.[10]

Therefore, the findings demonstrate the presence of a relationship of creativity with empathy, which is a low degree of correlation. The relationship of actualization with empathy is demonstrated by a moderate degree of correlation. The combination of creativity and actualization accounts for more variance than did either of the single correlations. Further, the difference between the larger single correlation and the multiple R is significant.

The findings of this study support the theoretical position proposed and, therefore, support the predictive ability of helicy. Since the variables chosen are proposed to be unitary manifestations of human beings and their relationships are based on the theoretical rationale of the Science of Unitary Human Beings, the findings suggest that human beings and environment do change together as postulated in helicy. The correlation coefficients and the percentage of covariance they share illustrates the support of the hypotheses in Table 13–2.

Because only 21 percent of the variance in empathy was accounted for, it is suggested that other variables characteristic of helicy be considered in future studies. One possible variable could be differentiation. Ference defined differentiation as increasing complexity and diversity and reported a 0.19 correlation with creativity.[4] Further, she suggested differentiation as a manifestation of unitary human development. Another possible variable could be mystical experience. Maslow suggested a relationship between mystical experience and self-actualization; this was tested by Hood, who reported a positive correlation.[14, 18]

DISCUSSION AND RECOMMENDATIONS

This study investigated the relationships of creativity, actualization, and empathy as constructs of human field pattern manifestations of the theoretical principle of helicy. Further, the study explored the adequacy of the instruments as measures of the constructs in the Science of Unitary Human Beings. The relationships among the variables tested the principle of helicy and provide a descriptive basis for further empirical investigation of the principle of helicy.

Helicy, postulated by Rogers, suggests that the nature and direction of unitary human development is continuously innovative and characterized by diversity of field pattern in relation to the continuous, mutual process between human and environmental fields.[23] The findings of this beginning descriptive study support Rogers' postulation of helicy as a principle of the nature and direction of unitary human development. Further, it supports the following recommendations for studies in the Science of Unitary Human Beings:

1. Creativity, actualization and empathy should be studied in relation to other possible manifestations of helicy because only 21 percent of the variance in empathy was accounted for by the combined independent variables
2. Replication should be carried out with a similar sample as well as with the following differences in the sample. A sample that has the same age range and participates in various religions should be considered because the sample frame represented a particular Protestant religious group. A sample of persons that included ages above 60 could further demonstrate the lack of significant differences in various age groups for the measures used. Lastly, the question has been raised as to whether the same manifestations would

be evident in non-Christian persons as were evident with the current sample. This question should be tested

3. Finally, the three tests used in this study should be validated through further use in the Science of Unitary Human Beings. This beginning descriptive study introduced these instruments in the science. These measures from the related disciplines may be useful as a guide for the development of tools to measure manifestations of unitary human development

REFERENCES

1. Crutchfield RS: The creative process. In Bloomberg M (ed): Creativity Theory and Research. New Haven, College & University Press, 1973
2. Damm VJ: Overall measures of self-actualization derived from the personal orientation inventory. Ed Psych Measure 29:977–981, 1969
3. Damm, VJ: Overall measures of self-actualization derived from the personal orientation inventory: A replication and refinement study. Ed Psych Measure 32:485–489, 1972
4. Ference HM: The Relationship of Time Experience, Creativity Traits, Differentiation and Human Field Motion, doctoral dissertation. New York University, 1979 (University Microfilms Publication No: 80-10, 281)
5. Fischer J: The validity of the personal orientation inventory for measuring the effects of training. Ed Psych Measure 37:1069–1074, 1977
6. Foster FP: The human relationships of creative individuals. J Creative Behav 2:111–118, 1968
7. Hogan R: Development of an empathy scale. J Consult Clin Psychol 33:307–316, 1969
8. Hood RW: Differential triggering of mystical experience as a function of self-actualization. Rev Relig Res 18:264–270, 1977
9. Koestler A: The Act of Creation. London, Hutchinson, 1964
10. Land GTL: Grow or Die. New York, Dell, 1973
11. Lash TV: Zen meditation and the development of empathy in counselors. J Humanistic Psych 10:39–74, 1970
12. Maslow A: Motivation and Personality, 2nd ed. New York, Harper & Row, Pub, 1954
13. Maslow A: The Psychology of Science. Chicago, Regnery, 1966
14. Maslow A: The Farther Reaches of Human Nature. New York, Viking, 1971
15. Mathes EW: Self-actualization, metavalues, and creativity. Psychol Rep 43:215–222, 1978
16. May R: The Courage to Create. New York, Norton, 1975
17. Murphy JP, Dauw D, Horton RE, et al.: Self-actualization and creativity. J Creative Behav 10:39–44, 1976
18. Nie N, Hull C, Jenkins J, et al.: Statistical Package for the Social Sciences, 2nd ed. New York, McGraw-Hill, 1975
19. Pearson PH, Maddi SR: The similes preference inventory: Development of a structured measure of the tendency toward variety. J Consult Psychol 30:301–308, 1966
20. Raile M: The Relationships of Creativity, Actualization, and Empathy in Unitary Human Development: A Descriptive Study of Rogers' Principle of Helicy, doctoral dissertation. New York University, 1983 (University Microfilms Publication No. 83-13, 874)
21. Rodriguez, AM: The Relationship Between a Measure of Self-Actualization and the

Facilitative Conditions Offered in Counseling, doctoral dissertation. University of Houston, 1977

22. Rogers C: A Way of Being. Boston, Houghton Mifflin, 1980
23. Rogers M: A science of unitary man. In Riehl JP, Roy C (eds): Conceptual Models for Nursing Practice, 2nd ed. New York, Appleton-Century-Crofts, 1980
24. Shostrom EL: An inventory for the measurement of self-actualization. Ed Psych Measure 14:207, 1964
25. Taylor IA: Empathic communication through nonverbal symbols in creative and noncreative subjects. Am Psychol 19:545, 1964
26. Taylor IA: An emerging view of creative actions. In Taylor IA and Getzels JW (eds): Perspectives in Creativity. Chicago, Aldine, 1975
27. Vargiu J: The purposeful imagination: Creativity. Synthesis, 3–4, 17–53, 1974

Critique of Alligood's Study

Joyce J. Fitzpatrick

Alligood studied the relationships of creativity and actualization to empathy as a test of Rogers' principle of helicy. She proposed creativity as a manifestation of innovation, actualization as a manifestation of increasing diversity, and empathy as another human field pattern of helicy. Thus, it was less clearly stated how empathy was specifically linked to Rogers' conceptualization. Alligood provided beginning detail regarding the derivation of the theoretical relationships. She provided some supporting literature from the work of Maslow and Carl Rogers, although this was not specifically integrated with her understanding of the Science of Unitary Human Beings.

A major strength of Alligood's study was her contribution to previous research. Some of the same variables were further explored. Alligood tied her research to that of Ference. It can also be related theoretically to the research of Cowling. Another strength of this study is the sample size. An avenue for future evaluation that is recommended is that of meta-analysis of these studies.

Like some of the previous studies, Alligood's would have benefited from a more rigorous methodology. She chose three self-report measures and could have provided data on which to assess the psychometric properties of the instruments. Alligood did not make the argument, for example, that these instruments, developed from different theoretical perspectives, were valid measures of the concepts within Rogers' model. Even if the choice had been made not to develop new measures, it might have been more advantageous here to include multiple measures, not only to assess validity, but also to explore the multidimensional nature of the variables.

Alligood also raised several questions for future exploration. As each of these projects represented an exploratory study related to Rogers' conceptualization, it is suggested that some collaborative future endeavors should occur.

Response

Martha Raile Alligood

I appreciate Fitzpatrick's critique of the chapter report of my study, and I am grateful for this opportunity to respond. Fitzpatrick's comments cluster around three areas, and I will address each area in the following order: (1) the theoretical rationale for the study: (2) the strengths of the study; and (3) the methodology of the study, including the rationale for tool selection.

The theoretical rationale for the study and, therefore, for the relationships tested in the study, derived directly from the principle of helicy as it is stated by Rogers. Helicy describes the nature and direction of human development as continuously innovative and characterized by diversity of field pattern in relation to the continuous mutual process of human and environmental fields.[2] In order to test helicy, it was necessary to identify field pattern manifestations that could be proposed as characteristic of helicy. Therefore, from the principle, the two characteristics of innovativeness and diversity of field pattern were identified. These characteristics are suggested by Rogers to emerge in relation to the continuous, mutual process of the human and environmental fields. Thus, the continuous, mutual process of the human and environmental fields was conceptualized as another characteristic of helicy. After intense study of these characteristics and extensive literature review, the following were identified as measurable unitary manifestations of the field pattern process. Creativity was proposed as a manifestation of innovativeness of field pattern; actualization was proposed as a manifestation of increasing diversity of field pattern; and empathy was proposed as a manifestation of the continuous, mutual process of the human–environment field pattern.

The theoretical relationships of these field pattern manifestations are derived directly from the relationships set forth by Rogers in the principle. That is, creativity will always be present as a manifestation of the continuous innovativeness of human development, as will actualization be a manifestation of the diversity of field pattern that is characteristic of development. These two characteristics, which I conceptualized as independent variables, emerge in relation to the continuous, mutual process (interaction) of human and environmental fields. I proposed empathy as a manifestation of the human and environment process and the dependent variable in relation to the emerging characteristics. Further, the positive relationships among the variables as hypothesized provided for testing the direction as well as the nature of the relationships theoretically proposed by helicy.

Therefore, the theoretical rationale for the study of the relationships was exclusively Rogers' conceptual system and specifically the principle of helicy. Maslow, Carl Rogers, and others were reviewed as related literature. Support of the relationships or lack of support was noted as it occurred in the related literature. However, it is keenly important to understand that the related literature was not included in the theoretical rationale for the study. Literature from other disciplines was related to the study because the variables under study were concepts developed from their English usage, and they were not unique to nursing.

Secondly, Fitzpatrick speaks to the strengths of the study. She mentions its connection to previous research. In addition, this study is one of several contemporary studies (including Cowling's research) that are based upon Rogers' theoretically and could, therefore, be related to the work of Ference. Fitzpatrick's suggestion for meta-analysis of these studies would certainly contribute to the development of the Science of Unitary Human Beings.

Another strength she cites is the sample size of 236 participants. Probably the greatest importance of the sample size is its contribution to the stability of the correlation coefficients. The support of each of the three hypotheses is strengthened by the significance $p < 0.001$, which contributes to the statistical power of probability.

Fitzpatrick's final point of discussion is the methodology and tool selection. Perhaps the greatest challenge researchers experience conducting studies to test the Science of Unitary Human Beings is that of measurement. Whereas some may choose to develop tools to measure the variables, others have felt the need to conduct descriptive studies to operationalize the abstract concepts. The latter is true of this researcher, and it is suggested that the findings from these descriptive studies will provide the base for tool development as well as further research.

At the time of this study and until the base is established, measures from other disciplines may be useful to studies in the Science of Unitary Human Beings. The uniqueness of the nursing perspective is demonstrated not only in the way a variable is measured but also in the selection of variables and in proposing their relationships. The latter two, selection of variables and proposing relationships, is seemingly more important at this beginning time, because that knowledge contributes to the basis for tool development. Ideas already presented in the discussion of the first two points in the critique provide further rationale for the tool selection in the present study.

The variables for the present study were identified as unitary manifestations of field pattern. These manifestations are measurable evidence of the characteristic of helicy suggested by the statement of the principle. As noted earlier, the variables were concepts not unique to nursing, and their definitions within the conceptual system were based on their English-usage definitions. Therefore, studies designed using variables whose definitions are true to the English-usage definition should be measurable with tools from other disciplines. Dagenais and Meleis[1] propose this as an alternative in tool selection. Presumably these measures may not be as precise as those designed within the conceptual system. However, they should capture the essence of the variable if the sample size is sufficient—which leads further to the rationale for the design of this study using tools from other disciplines.

The large sample size has already been identified by Fitzpatrick as a strength of the study. In a study where measurement of relationships among variables is proposed as evidence of support for a principle that theoretically predicted the relationships, the stability of the correlation coefficients becomes increasingly important. The stability of the correlation coefficient contributes to the statistical power of their probability. The stability is a product of the statistical significance. The large sample size with a small number of variables yielded correlation coefficients $p < 0.001$. This stability is especially important in light of the previous discussion of measurement with tools developed in other disciplines.

The critique has provided three main areas of discussion and has afforded me the opportunity to respond and further clarify regarding the theoretical rationale, the strengths, and the methodology of my study. The points raised have challenged me to explain further the rationale for decisions made in the process. I have appreciated the opportunity.

REFERENCES

1. Dagenais F, Meleis A: Professionalism, work ethic, and empathy in nursing: The nurse self-description form. West J Nurs Res 4:407–422, 1982
2. Rogers, ME: A science of unitary man. In Riehl JP, Roy C (eds): Conceptual Models for Nursing Practice, 2nd ed. New York, Appleton-Century-Crofts, 1980

Critique of Alligood's Study

Violet M. Malinski

Alligood explored creativity, actualization, and empathy as possible manifestations of helicy. Because the mutual process of unitary humans and environment is the phenomenon of concern in this system, she framed an appropriate problem for study within the Science of Unitary Human Beings. In addition to testing for helicy in developing individuals, which contributes to the evolution of the system, this descriptive study makes a further contribution by explicating the "development" of individuals as described by the principle of helicy as proposed by Rogers.

Alligood presented an overview of the derivation of the variables selected for study as they related to characteristics of field patterning as proposed by Rogers. Background literature, although briefly cited, was highlighted to demonstrate support for proposed relationships and to indicate that the relationships hypothesized among the three variables under study were novel ones not previously explored.

Rather than develop new measures, Alligood chose to use tests previously developed, exploring their potential for use in studies of unitary humans. Whereas Ference employed the Adjective Check List to assess creativity, Alligood used the Similes Preference Inventory, thus providing data on a second tool for researchers to consider and continue to test for applicability within this system. Toward this end, it would have been useful if she had shared data on reliability and validity from this and from other investigations.

Although she was not able to sample randomly, Alligood did collect data from a large number of subjects. It is interesting that she chose to start with a Christian sample, recommending that the study be replicated with a non-Christian one. It is not clear that this differentiation has validity within the system under study.

Alligood found support for her hypotheses, although only a moderate correlation for the relationship of creativity and actualization, taken together, with empathy. In a sense, this treatment of the variables could be interpreted as an attempt to differentiate helicy into "component parts," which would be incompatible with this framework. Therefore, as well as pursuing the directions proposed by Alligood for future research, it might be advantageous to explore the principles together as manifested by the correlates of patterning as an option to testing the principles separately as a base for continuing the study of this system.

Alligood clearly identified her research as a beginning, descriptive study. She has contributed to the formation of a base on which future researchers can draw in determining directions for their own work.

Response
Martha Raile Alligood

I appreciate this opportunity to respond to the critique of my study written by Malinski. Because Rogers has said the principles of homeodynamics postulate the nature and direction of developmental change, it follows that the measurement of manifestations of pattern, especially those which Rogers includes as characteristics of helicy, should provide evidence of helicy being operational or evident in developing individuals. These manifestations of helicy should be present in all individuals and are not measuring development per se, but characteristics of unitary human development. With regard to the statement that the phenomenon of concern is unitary human beings and environment, within Rogers' system, when we measure the human beings, we are at the same time measuring their environment because of integrality.

Secondly, the matter of measurement within the system will be addressed. As Malinski noted, this beginning descriptive study was carried out using measures or tools that were developed in other disciplines. I would suggest that, at least for the present time in the Science of Unitary Human Beings, the measures from other disciplines may be useful to us. This is suggested especially in beginning descriptive studies. The uniqueness of the nursing perspective in our discipline is not only the way in which the variable is measured, but also it is the selection of the variables and their proposed relationships that are more important because they provide a basis for tool development. Studies designed with variables whose definitions are true to the English-language definitions should be measurable with tools from various disciplines. Presumably these measures would not be as precise as those designed within the conceptual system, but they should capture the essence of the variable if the sample size is large enough to provide a stable measurement. The sample size of 236 in a study with three variables provided correlation coefficients significant at $p < 0.001$, which is a very stable measure. This has been noted as a strong point of the study.

Thirdly, Malinski suggests that information on reliability and validity of the instruments would be useful. Each of the measures used in this study had been used and reliability and validity reported in the literature. The Similes Preference Inventory had reported Kuder-Richardson 20 values of 0.95, 0.95, and 0.93 in three different studies to establish internal consistency.[4] Construct validity was established using the convergent-type process. In the present study the Kuder-Richardson 21 formula was used, and the reliability coefficient of 0.80 was computed.

The Personal Orientation Inventory is the most widely used and published measure of actualization. The I-scale was used as a single measure of actualization based on the work of Damm, Hood, and Yonge.[1-3, 5] The reported reliability coefficient was 0.77. In the present study, a reliability coefficient of 0.70 was computed.

The Hogan Scale was reported in the literature with coefficients ranging from 0.52 to 0.77. In the present study the reliability coefficient was computed at 0.50. Although this coefficient was lower than desired, the large sample size contributed to reliability, and the index of reliability was computed at 0.70, which is acceptable.

Malinski's fourth point regarding the sample frame is well taken. Persons' religious affiliation or religiosity in general is irrelevant in the conceptual system. In fact, the means and standard deviations on each measure were congruent with those reported in the literature. However, because the question is often raised with regard to the sample, I suggested the study could be conducted with several different samples and, particularly, one without religious preference. This is a methodology question and not a theoretical one, to be sure.

Regarding Malinski's fifth point concerning the possibility of viewing the variables as "parts" of helicy, Rogers has included within the principle of helicy the manifestations that were measured, that is: innovative as creative, more diverse as actualized, and human–environmental integrality as empathy. The identification of behavioral manifestations of the pattern in no way is suggesting component parts. There are identifiable pattern manifestations we call behaviors and feelings, which manifest the unitary human being. This study took Rogers' principle of helicy and the behaviors she has alluded to in the principle to begin to see if this principle is operational in human beings. The principle of integrality was included in this study. Rogers says integrality is subsumed in helicy. The measurement of empathy in the present study was a manifestation of integrality, strictly speaking. The principle of resonancy has been tested or is being tested. I would suggest that with the baseline information from this and other beginning descriptive studies, broader studies can be designed. I would caution, however, that the testing of the framework will be in the measurement of principles and theories derived from the system, and these studies will be developed assuming the conceptual system for study. The total conceptual system cannot be tested because it is assumed and provides the basis for principles and theories that are being derived.

I want to thank Malinski for her critique, which has challenged my ideas and led me to clarify or explain rationale. This exercise has led me to re-examine the way in which my work fits in the larger context of Rogers' Science of Unitary Human Beings. If this dialogue will assist others in understanding the work that has been done in the system, perhaps it will also assist in the development of further studies. That is my professional goal in presenting my work.

REFERENCES

1. Damm VJ: Overall measures of self-actualization derived from the personal orientation inventory. Ed Psych Measure 29:977–981, 1969
2. Damm VJ: Overall measures of self-actualization derived from the personal orientation inventory: A replication and refinement study. Ed Psych Measure 32:485–489, 1972
3. Hood RW: Differential triggering of mystical experience as a function of self-actualization. Rev Relig Res 18:264–310, 1977
4. Pearson PH, Maddi SR: The similes preference inventory: Development of a structured measure of the tendency toward variety. J Consult Psychol 30:301–308, 1966
5. Yonge GD: Time experience, self-actualization values, and creativity. J Pers Assess 39:601–606, 1975

14

The Relationship Between Imposed Motion and Human Field Motion in Elderly Individuals Living in Nursing Homes

Sarah Hall Gueldner

The primary purpose of this study was to test empirically Rogers' conceptual system by describing the relationship that exists between imposed motion (rocking) and human field motion. A secondary purpose was to determine if perceived human field motion is correlated with perceived restedness. The quasi-experimental design consisted of a 5-day control regimen followed by a 5-day treatment regimen. The treatment consisted of 10-minute periods of rocking at a prescribed rate each day for 5 consecutive days. Group 1 ($N = 10$) rocked at their individually preferred rates; Group 2 ($N = 13$) rocked at the imposed rate of 34–36 rocking cycles per minute; and Group 3 ($N = 8$), serving as the control group, sat without rocking in mechanically immobilized rocking chairs throughout each treatment session. Ference's Human Field Motion Test (HFMT) and Smith's Restedness–Tiredness Scale (RTS) were used to measure the dependent variables of human field motion and restedness, respectively. Each subject was tested prior to the control regimen, between the control and treatment regimens, and following the treatment regimen. The sample consisted of 31 mentally alert and ambulatory nursing home residents 60 to 93 years of age. Analysis of variance procedures did not demonstrate a statistically significant difference ($p = 0.05$) between the absolute post-treatment HFMT scores of the subjects who rocked and those control subjects who did not rock. However, 77 percent of those subjects who rocked at an imposed rate manifested increased post-treatment HFMT scores, while only 23 percent of the nonrocking control subjects reported increasing post-treatment HFMT scores. This seeming proportional trend would suggest that a relationship could possibly be

161

demonstrated between human field motion and rocking under a more intensive treatment regimen. The HFMT scores and RTS were negatively correlated ($p = 0.01$) using Pearson's correlation coefficients, indicating that subjects reporting higher human field motion also felt more rested.

BACKGROUND: GENESIS OF PROBLEM FORMULATION

The concept of fatigue was originally selected for investigation in this study because it is a phenomenon often associated with perceived well-being. Although the literature revealed numerous characteristics relative to the nature of fatigue, it was soon evident that the concept has not yet been defined in a way consistent with the Rogerian conceptual system, which demands a unitary definition rather than a definition of parts. Although environment and movement, concepts central to the Rogerian system, were repeatedly studied in connection with the phenomenon of fatigue, fatigue is itself defined in the literature in terms of subjective and physical components. [1-3, 7, 8, 11, 13, 14, 18, 19, 26, 27, 33]

The myriad of specific physical and subjective manifestations attributed to fatigue would seem to suggest that it is, in fact, a unitary phenomenon manifested by the human energy field for which there is a wide range of indices. Indeed, the possibility exists that the multifaceted phenomena collectively described as fatigue are merely manifestations of the condition of an individual's human energy field and reveal the relative motion within that field. Based on this logic, the focus of this study became centered on the basic nature of the human energy field. Because study of the human energy field is still in early stages, it was believed that additional basic theoretical investigation must preface primary study of manifestations and expressions of the energy field such as fatigue. The basic concept under investigation in this study was further restricted to the phenomenon described by Rogers and Ference as human field motion. [9, 23]

In keeping with earlier research interests of the investigator, an elderly population provided the sample for this study. Based on review of the gerontological literature, which repeatedly addressed the particular importance of movement in the care and well-being of the aged, a program of regular, imposed motion (rocking) was designed as the treatment condition to be tested in this study. [5, 6, 12, 16, 17]

RELATIONSHIP TO THE SCIENCE OF UNITARY HUMAN BEINGS

Because it purports to study the possibility of variations in the human energy field, this investigation flows directly from the philosophy, assumptions, and principles of Rogers' Science of Unitary Human Beings. [23] The postulate of Rogers' system relating most directly to the study of the relationship of imposed motion to human field motion is the principle of resonancy. The principle states that "the human field and environmental field are identified by wave patterns manifesting continuous change from lower frequency waves to higher frequency waves." [25] This principle provides justification for the use of Ference's Human Field Motion Test (HFMT), which purports to measure relative states of human field motion through a series of semantic differential scales judged to elicit responses ranging from lower to high wave frequency.[9] The principle of resonancy in fact will be tested directly under the treatment condition of imposed motion. While not directly tested during this study, Rogers' principles of helicy and integrality are postulated to explain the nature of the human–environment interaction under investigation.

In keeping with the philosophy of acausality crucial to the Rogerian system, the three hypotheses posited to guide this research were stated in terms of postulated relationships rather than in statements of implied causality. They are as follows:

1. A positive relationship exists between imposed motion (rocking) and perceived human field motion in elderly individuals residing in nursing homes. Nursing home residents who rock will manifest higher post-treatment HFMT scores than will the control subjects who do not rock
2. A stronger positive relationship exists between preferred rate of rocking and perceived human field motion than between imposed rate of rocking and perceived human field motion. Those subjects allowed to rock at their preferred rates will manifest greater perceived human field motion than will those who are forced to rock at an imposed rate
3. A positive relationship exists between perceived human field motion and reported level of restedness, as measured by Smith's Restedness–Tiredness Scale

METHOD

This study was conducted within three privately owned nursing homes located in a rural area of the southeastern United States. The nursing homes had bed capacities of 100, 178, and 76, respectively. Approximately 13 percent of the residents were private-paying.

The sample for this study consisted of 31 individuals who had lived in the nursing home for at least 1 month prior to data collection and who were (1) 60 years of age or older; (2) ambulatory; (3) sighted; (4) English-speaking; and (5) mentally alert as determined by Pfeiffer's[20] Short Portable Mental Status Questionnaire (SPMSQ). Only those individuals who expressed a willingness to participate were included in the study.

Of the 31 subjects completing the study, most were Caucasian (87 percent), female (75 percent), 70 years of age or older (81 percent), and had not completed high school (86 percent). Of the subjects, 58 percent ambulated without assisting devices; 26 percent required wheelchairs for ambulation part or all of the time; and 16 percent used canes or walkers during ambulation at least part of the time.

Sample recruitment and retention posed a continuing problem to this investigation. Out of a total of 102 individuals identified by the nursing home staff as potential subjects, only 56 met the criteria and began the study protocol. Eighteen of those approached by the investigator declined the invitation to participate, 4 citing fear that the rocking would aggravate chronic episodes of dizziness. Twenty-two of the potential subjects were excluded because of insufficient scores on Pfeiffer's Short Portable Mental Status Questionnaire, and two others were excluded because of insurmountable hearing problems.

Of the 56 nursing home residents who began the protocol, only 31 completed all treatment and testing sessions. Most absences were due to physical complaints (45 percent); of these, 3 gave dizziness as the reason for their absence. Conflicting appointments accounted for the remaining absences from treatment sessions.

A quasiexperimental design was implemented in this study. Subjects from each nursing home were randomly assigned to one of two experimental groups (Groups 1 or 2) or to the control group (Group 3). The study design provided data that could be examined for possible correlations among the dependent variables of human field motion and restedness, the independent variable of imposed motion, the extraneous variable of socialization, and selected demographic variables.

A modified form of Ference's HFMT served as the primary measurement tool for this study. Ference reported the reliability index of the scale-concept sets to be 0.87 during reliability testing in 1979. Retest reliability was found to be 0.77 in 1978 testings and 0.70 in 1979. These reliability data were obtained from a sample of 213 subjects who were from 30 to 60 years of age. Additional information concerning validity and development of the tool may be found in Chapter 9.

During a preliminary survey, several potential problems emerged relative to the use of this tool with the particular population selected for this study. For instance, the average level of formal education reported by the 16 elderly individuals in the pilot survey was less than the sixth-grade level. In contrast, the HFMT was validated almost exclusively with a highly educated sample, and some terms used in it were judged to require a higher reading level than was characteristic of the potential subjects in this study.[30, 32]

To more fully assess the anticipated problem, items listed on the original HFMT were read as written to 10 randomly selected individuals 60 years old or older, and each individual was asked to describe what the terms meant. Ninety percent of the pilot subjects were unfamiliar with at least one term in the *pragmatic–visionary* descriptor set, and 60 percent had considerable difficulty comprehending the meanings of the terms *propel, finite,* and *transcendent.* To a lesser degree, the terms *boundaryless, passive, imaginative,* and *unimaginative* posed a recognition problem to pilot subjects.

Because it has been established that up to three of the scales may be deleted without altering the validity and reliability of the tool, the *pragmatic–visionary* descriptor set was deleted for use with this population.[10] The decision was made to retain all other descriptor sets in the test and to offer substitute words when necessary to assist the subjects to understand a term.

In addition to recognition problems, a preliminary study conducted by the investigator with a similar population revealed that vision problems and limited experience with questionnaires made it difficult for many elderly individuals to record accurate written responses without assistance. Just being asked to respond to a written questionnaire seemed to constitute a source of stress for some subjects. In light of these observations, the HFMT was administered to each subject separately, in an interview-type setting. The bipolar descriptors, printed in 1-inch black letters were displayed one set at a time at opposite ends of a heavy seven-sectioned line similar to those printed on Ference's tool. Each subject was asked to place his or her finger on the line at the point that best represented his or her self-perception with regard to each set of descriptors. The numerical value of each response, as determined by the guidelines accompanying the HFMT, was then recorded. The scale is designed so that a high score on the HFMT indicates a state of increased human field motion.

As interest in the concept of fatigue was the original inspiration for this study, Smith's Restedness–Tiredness Scale was utilized as a secondary measuring device in an attempt to demonstrate a relationship between human field motion and reported expressions of restedness–tiredness.[28, 29] This tool is a modification of Borg's Rating Scale of Perceived Exertion, which has a reliability of 0.83.[4] Smith administered the modified tool to 180 male and female subjects between the ages of 18 and 35 years in an effort to determine the relationship of restedness and/or tiredness to a variety of environmental settings. A reliability coefficient of 0.67 was reported between the ratings of two consecutive mornings for subjects who had just awakened. In keeping with the previously established characteristics of the population, a large display board with 1-inch black letters and numbers was used to administer this instrument to each subject. Lower scores on the RTS indicate perceived restedness (less fatigue), while high scores indicate perceived tiredness (more fatigue).

Five-Day Control Regimen

A 5-day control regimen was included in the study to control for the introduction of members of the research team into the subject's environment and for the socialization that occurred as the residents sat together in newly formed groups. Starting on the Monday immediately following completion of the initial interviews and pretesting sessions, each group of subjects (Group 1, 2, and 3 in each nursing home) came to the preselected dayroom and sat in regular chairs for 10 minutes each day for 5 consecutive days. A bell timer signaled the end of each session. Four to six members of the research team sat or stood in the room throughout each session. During the first session, the investigator explained that conversation would be limited as part of the study protocol.

Five-Day Experimental Regimen

The treatment applied in this investigation consisted of periods of imposed motion in the form of (1) rocking at each subject's preferred rate, (2) rocking at an imposed rate, or (3) sitting in a rocker without rocking. Since research related to the concept of human field motion is still developmental in nature, search of the literature did not reveal an established relationship between the frequency and duration of imposed motion and change in human field motion. Therefore, a treatment regimen of one 10-minute session daily for 5 consecutive days was selected as the treatment condition for this beginning investigative endeavor. This period of time was selected because it was believed to be of sufficient duration to test the hypotheses without requiring undue exertion on the part of any subject.

Treatment Regimen I (Preferred Rate)

Subjects assigned to Group 1 in each nursing home were asked to rock at their preferred rates during each treatment session. A research assistant stood behind each rocking chair for the entire 10-minute period and used a thumb-controlled event counter to obtain a numerical assessment of each subject's rocking cycles. The numerical sum of rocking cycles thus recorded was divided by 10 to obtain the rocking rate for each subject during each rocking session.

Treatment Regimen II (Imposed Rate)

Subjects in Group 2 at each nursing home were asked to rock at a rate of 35 backward-forward cycles per minute during each treatment session. An electric metronome was used as a guide for the rate. A variance of plus or minus one rocking cycle per minute was accepted. Again, a research assistant stood behind each rocking chair and used a thumb-controlled event counter to verify that the imposed rate was being maintained. If a subject was unable to rock at the specified rate, the assigned research assistant, holding only the back of the rocker, instituted the prescribed rate for the duration of the session.

Treatment Regimen III (Nonrocking Control)

After the research team had immobilized each rocking chair by placing a wooden wedge under each rocker, subjects in Group 3 were asked to sit in the rocking chairs during each treatment session.

RESULTS

Analysis of variance based on a repeated measures design was used as the statistical technique to test hypotheses 1 and 2. This technique is a regression procedure designed to identify significant interactions between the dependent variable (HFMT), the treatment groups, and time of testing. No statistically significant main or interactive effects were demonstrated between treatment groups relative to scores on HFMT I, II, or III. No significant difference was found in the HFMT scores between subjects who rocked and those who did not rock, nor was significant difference found between the HFMT scores of subjects who rocked at their preferred rates and those who rocked at the imposed rate. Hypotheses 1 and 2 were therefore rejected.

Pearson correlation coefficients were obtained to test hypothesis 3. When treatment groups were collapsed to form one group, a statistically significant ($p = 0.01$) negative relationship was demonstrated between HFMT scores and RTS scores, indicating that subjects who expressed feelings of high human field motion also reported feeling a high degree of restedness (Table 14–1). Accordingly, hypothesis 3 was retained.

Although no statistically significant differences in absolute HFMT scores were demonstrated between groups, perusal of the raw data revealed that a larger percentage of subjects who rocked (Groups 1 and 2) manifested increased scores on HFMT III than did the nonrocking subjects in the control group (Group 3). A histographic presentation of this finding is provided in Figure 14–1.

A statistically significant relationship was demonstrated between reported goodness of sleep and scores on both HFMT III and RTS III. No statistically significant differences were identified for the HFMT or RTS scores relative to age; sex; level of education; status of mobility; or ingestion of tranquilizers, antidepressants, or sedatives–hypnotics.

The Cronbach-Alpha reliability coefficient was found to be 0.76 for the "motor is running" scale of the HFMT, 0.74 for the "field expansion" scale, and 0.84 overall. The *finite–transcendent* word pair was reported to be unfamiliar by 92 percent of the original 56 subjects in the study group, and 23 percent did not know the meaning of the *imaginative–unimaginative* descriptor pair. To a lesser degree, recognition problems were observed wtih the *continuous–discontinuous, active–passive, drag–propel, and boundaryless–limited* descriptor sets.

DISCUSSION AND RECOMMENDATIONS

Because no significant differences in the absolute HFMT scores were isolated with regard to treatment groups and testing sessions, one must conclude that no statistically significant relationship existed between rocking and human field motion in this study. However, this finding would not rule out the possibility that a relationship may exist between rocking and perceived human field motion in other sam-

TABLE 14–1. SUMMARY OF PEARSON CORRELATION COEFFICIENTS FOR HFMT SCORES WITH RTS SCORES FOR COLLAPSED GROUPS BY TESTING SESSION

Testing Session	Coefficient*
HFMT I/RTS I	−0.48
HFMT II/RTS II	−0.58
HFMT III/RTS III	−0.48

*$p < 0.01$.

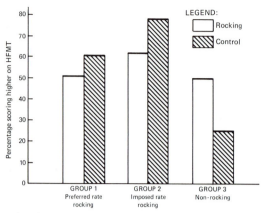

Figure 14–1. Proportional comparison of subjects, by group, scoring higher on HFMT following contol and rocking regimes.

ples or with other types of imposed motion. It is also possible that the treatment regimen implemented in this study was not of sufficient strength or duration to expose a measurable relationship between rocking and field motion. The likelihood of this possibility is increased by the observation that a greater percentage of subjects who rocked had increased post-treatment HFMT scores than did subjects who did not rock. The inability to demonstrate a relationship could also be associated with the small number of subjects completing the study protocol. The statistical management of the data was hindered by both the small sample size and the resulting unequal cell sizes. Finally, since instrument development for the concept of human field motion is just beginning, it is also possible that the instrument of measurement used in this investigation lacks the necessary sensitivity to verify such a relationship in this sample.

This investigator therefore would contend that investigation of the relationship between human field motion and imposed motion be rigorously continued and expanded, as documentation of this relationship seems particularly germane to the validation of Rogers' conceptual system.

The findings of this research have also raised other significant questions regarding the relationship that exists among human field motion, sleep patterns, and perceived restedness, which hold relevance for future study as well as for practice. A statistically significant positive relationship was demonstrated between perceived human field motion and restedness, and goodness of sleep was found to be positively correlated with both human field motion and perceived restedness. These associations suggest that the phenomena of fatigue and decreased human field motion may share common characteristics. Because fatigue has been repeatedly linked with slowed recovery and predisposition to poor health, increased study is needed to establish the more complete nature of these relationships as a possible basis for nursing action.

Implementation of the treatment regimen in this study also pointed out the need for development of a mechanized rocking device that could be set at a constant rocking rate. Such a device would increase standardization of the treatment condition and reduce the number of research assistants needed to conduct the study. For similar reasons, it would be advantageous to modify the study design to reduce the number of subjects participating in the treatment at any one time. These modifications would greatly decrease the extraneous variable of socialization.

Although the unique characteristics identified in this sample cannot be generalized without further study of the broader nursing home population, the population-related challenges encountered during implementation of this study hold practical implications for nursing investigations involving similar populations. The characteristically low level of formal education, frequently compromised mobility, problems with vision and hearing, and relative inexperience with research instruments and protocols must be taken into account when selecting methods and instrumentation for use with institutionalized aged populations. Likewise, complaints of dizziness were found to be widespread (11 percent) within this population, a factor that tends to limit full randomness of representation of this group for study involving imposed motion.

In summary, the investigator offers the following recommendations for further research:

1. That the theoretical research effort related to the phenomenon of human field motion be continued and expanded, particularly as it is related to a variety of types of imposed motion and sleep patterns
2. That the HFMT be modified or a companion tool be developed for use with this and other populations who have less formal education than the individuals who participated in the development of the instrument
3. That future study involving rocking as a treatment condition be modified to include rocking sessions of longer duration
4. That a portion of future study involving rocking include other populations of varying ages, educational levels, and life-styles
5. That a mechanized rocking device be designed in order to standardize the treatment regime and reduce the size of the research team
6. That future research be designed to explore more fully the relationship that exists between perceived human field motion and perceived restedness–tiredness in similar and other populations
7. That future study involving similar populations be designed in such a way that fewer subjects participate in the control and treatment regimens at any one time
8. That future study be directed toward the more complete assessment of the incidence and description of the phenomenon of dizziness as it occurs in elderly populations
9. That future research efforts involving similar populations be modified so as to better accommodate out-of-building commitments, institutional schedules, and occasional disabling physical discomforts

REFERENCES

1. Akerstedt T, Palmblad J, de la Torre B, et al.: Adrenocortical and gonadal steroids during sleep deprivation. Sleep 3(1):23–29, 1980
2. Bartlett F: Psychological criteria of fatigue. In Floyd W, Welford A (eds): Symposium on Fatigue and Symposium on Human Factors in Equipment Design. New York, Arno Press, 1977
3. Bartley SH, Chute E: Fatigue and Impairment in Man. New York, McGraw-Hill, 1947
4. Borg GAV (ed): Physical Work and Effort. Oxford, Pergamon Press, 1977
5. Borgman MF: Exercise and health maintenance. J Nurs Ed 16(1):6, 1977
6. Burnside I: Working with the Elderly. North Scituate, Mass, Duxbury Press, 1978
7. Dana R: The Human Machine in Industry. Easton, Ill, Hive, 1980
8. Edholm O: Tropical fatigue. In Floyd W, Welford A (eds): Symposium on Fatigue and Symposium on Human Factors in Equipment Design. New York, Arno Press, 1977
9. Ference HM: The Relationship of Time Experience, Creativity Traits, Differentiation, and Human Field Motion, doctoral dissertation. New York University, 1979
10. Ference HM: Personal communication, May 1982
11. Glenville M: Effects of sleep deprivation on short-duration performance measures compared to the Auditory Vigilance Task. Sleep 1(2):129–176, 1978
12. Goldberg W, Fitzpatrick J: Movement therapy with the aged. Nurs Res 29:339–346, 1980
13. Goldmark J: Fatigue and efficiency. New York, Russell Sage Foundation, 1912
14. Grandjean E: Fatigue: Its physiological and psychological significance. Ergonomics 11:427–436, 1968
15. Gueldner S: Energy levels in the institutionalized aged. J Alabama Acad Sci 53(3):92, 1982
16. Laban T: The Mastery of Movement. Boston, Plays, Inc., 1971
17. Newman MA: Movement tempo and the experience of time. Nurs Res 25:273–279, 1976
18. Numeley SA, Dowd P, Myhre L, Stribley R: Physiological and psychological effects of heat stress simulating cockpit conditions. Aviat Space Environ Med 49:763–787, 1978
19. Opstad P, Ekanger R, Nummestad M, Raabe N: Performance, mood, and clinical symptoms in men exposed to prolonged, severe physical work and sleep deprivation. Aviation, Space, Environ Med 49:1065–1073, 1978
20. Pfeiffer E: A short, portable, mental status questionnaire for the assessment of organic brain deficit in elderly patients. J Am Geriatr Soc 23:433–441, 1975
21. Rogers M: An Introduction to the Theoretical Basis of Nursing. Philadelphia, FA Davis, 1970
22. Rogers ME: Science of unitary man: A paradigm for nursing. Paper presented at the International Congress of Applied Systems Research and Cybernetics, Acapulco, December 12–16, 1980
23. Rogers M: Science of unitary man: A paradigm for nursing. In Lasker GE (ed): Applied Systems and Cybernetics. New York, Pergamon Press, 1981
24. Rogers ME: Personal communication, 1982
25. Rogers ME: Principles of homeodynamics. New York University, 1982 (unpublished)
26. Schwabe RS: Motivation in measurements of fatigue. In Floyd W, Welford A (eds): Symposium on Fatigue and Symposium on Human Factors in Equipment Design. New York, Arno Press, 1977

27. Simonson E, Weiser P: Psychological Aspects and Physiological Correlates of Work and Fatigue. Springfield, Ill, Charles C Thomas, 1976
28. Smith MJ: The auditory environment and temporal experience as related to perceived energy for subjects confined to bed. Paper presented at the 1981 Annual Business and Program Meeting of the Council of Nurse Researchers, American Nurses' Association, Washington, D.C., September 16–19, 1981
29. Smith MJ: (faculty member, Morgantown University School of Nursing, Morgantown, WVa) Personal communication, February 8, 1982
30. South Carolina Word List—Grades 1–12. Los Angeles, Instructional Objectives Exchange, 1981
31. Statistical Abstracts of the United States (101st ed). Washington, D.C., U.S. Department of Commerce, Bureau of the Census, 1980
32. Thorndike E, Lorge I: The Teacher's Word Book of 30,000 Words. New York, Columbia University Teachers' College, Bureau of Publications, 1944
33. Weston HC: Visual fatigue. In Floyd W, Welford A (eds): Symposium on Fatigue and Symposium on Human Factors in Equipment Design. New York, Arno Press, 1977

Critique of Gueldner's Study

Joyce J. Fitzpatrick

Gueldner studied the relationships between imposed motion (rocking) and human field motion, and between human field motion and restedness. Her research was directly based on the work of other Rogers scholars. Such building of research can be beneficial in expanding both the understandings and the data base. It was not suggested with any of these studies that there will be an attempt to pool the data.

Conceptualizations that were central to this investigation included the principle of resonancy and the concept of human field motion. Gueldner also suggested that fatigue was central to her concerns. She proposed it as a manifestation of unitary persons. Gueldner did not, however, provide direct theoretical or empirical support for her postualtions. The explication of a relationship with rhythm theory would have been desired, and could be used to link the concepts and variables.

Gueldner's study included some methodological problems, e.g., small sample size. However, if framed as an experimental study, this research should lead to further related investigations. The investigator should continue to explore these relationships in more tightly designed research and more fully explicate the conceptual links to Rogers and the theoretical links among the variables.

An additional concern that Gueldner appropriately addressed was that lack of understanding of key test words among the cohort of elderly persons. Additional pilot testing of this human field motion test would be recommended, as this problem may also occur with persons in other age cohorts depending on educational preparation.

In summary, Gueldner's study represented a creative approach to investigation of phenomena of interest to Rogers. Gueldner has translated her concern for the well-being of older people into a research question that deserves additional attention.

Response
Sarah Hall Gueldner

I concur with the points of critique offered by Fitzpatrick and appreciate the suggestions offered for future investigations.

Fitzpatrick's suggestion that investigators studying concepts within the Rogerian system begin to pool data is an excellent one. Such a pool would particularly enhance the development and refinement of tools to measure the still elusive concepts within the system and would facilitate a more complete understanding of the relationships within the theory. Access to such a data pool from other studies using the Ference tool for measuring human field motion would perhaps provide a relatively quick way to determine if terms found to be problematic for subjects in this sample posed similar problems for samples in other investigations. It could further be established to what extent level of education was associated with the difficulties encountered. Since all tools presently being used to test the Rogerian system are still in developmental stages, such a data pool would greatly speed the process of tool development.

Development of such a data base pool would also offer a partial solution to the problem of small sample size noted by Fitzpatrick. Tests of a theoretical framework within a clinical setting have traditionally been fraught with difficulty recruiting and/or retaining a sample of sufficient size, particularly if the research involves a period of manipulation of a variable over time. For instance, while 56 subjects started this study, only 31 completed the study protocol. Certainly this high attrition rate was disappointing to me. But it is so crucial that theory be studied within the practice area that it seems nurse researchers may at times have to endure less than ideal sample sizes. Maintenance of a data pool would greatly improve the yield of the findings emerging from studies involving relatively small samples.

Finally, I acknowledge the weak theoretical link that was developed in this study between the conceptualization of fatigue and the Rogerian system. As discussed in the chapter, I plan to develop this theoretical link more fully in future investigations. Certainly rhythm theory will be central to this linkage. At this time, however, the definition of fatigue is itself too multifacted to link as a single concept to the Rogerian system.

15

Investigation of the Principle of Helicy: The Relationship of Human Field Motion and Power

Elizabeth Ann Manhart Barrett

Starting from the basis of Rogers' conceptual system, this investigator: (1) extended the system to describe the phenomenon of power as well as the interrelationship of concepts (awareness, choices, freedom to act intentionally, the involvement in creating changes) that represented manifestations of power; (2) developed an instrument to measure dimensions of the theoretical power construct; (3) devised a new method of analyzing and scoring the Human Field Motion Test; (4) designed and conducted reliability and construct validity studies.[1] Following two judges' studies and a pilot study ($N = 267$), the final study ($N = 625$) investigated the principle of helicy by testing the relationship between human field motion (HFM) measures, which represented the direction of change, and the power (P) measures, which represented the nature of change. It was hypothesized that there was at least one significant relationship between the set of HFM measures and the set of concepts-contexts-scales measuring power. Following factor analysis, factor scores were computed for the HFM and P data, and the hypothesis was tested utilizing canonical correlation design.

The hypothesis was supported with the sum of two statistically significant squared canonical correlations accounting for 40 percent of shared variance among the two sets of variables. This was interpreted as suggesting that as HFM, an index of unitary human development, proceeds, so does the human being's capacity to participate knowingly in the nature of that development. *Power* describes a way humans interact with their environment to actualize some developmental potentials rather than others and, thereby, share in the creation of reality.

BACKGROUND: GENESIS OF PROBLEM FORMULATION

Derived from Rogers'[38] conceptual system and, specifically, the principle of helicy, this power theory endorsed mutual, simultaneous processes and questioned causality, domination, and control. The theoretical formulation utilized concepts from relevant literature, such as intentionality and will, and related them to themes from the power literature. However, it was the interrelation of the concepts as manifestations of power from a nursing science viewpoint that was different from the diverse theoretical perspectives, often based on closed-system models, presented in the literature. The theory was derived specifically from the principle of helicy and explicated the relationship of measures indicative of the direction of change (human field motion variables) and measures indicative of the nature of change (power variables). Hence, selected characteristics of the human field pattern were operationalized as empirical indicants of human change.

RELATIONSHIP TO THE SCIENCE OF UNITARY HUMAN BEINGS

Helicy concerns the nature and direction of change.[39] While Rogers does not discuss power, her notion that humans can knowingly participate in change linked the principle of helicy to development of a power theory consistent with the assumptions, building blocks, and principles of Rogers' conceptual system. The theory conceptualized human field motion as an indicator of the direction of change, i.e., a change in position, and power as an indicator of the nature of change, i.e., a change in participation. It was hypothesized that human field motion and power would be related. It had been suggested by previous research that human field motion is an index of unitary human development,[9] and it was postulated that power is the way humans participate in the nature of that development.

Power was defined as the capacity to participate knowingly in the nature of change characterizing the continuous repatterning of the human and environmental fields. Power is being aware of what one is choosing to do, feeling free to do it, and doing it intentionally. Depending on the nature of the awareness, the choices one makes, and the freedom to act intentionally, the range of situations in which one is involved in creating change varies.

Power is a relative state characterized by the momentary continuously changing pattern; power is also a relative trait characterized by the more consistent organization of the human and environmental field pattern. Power is felt, cognizant activity that can manifest in a variety of forms. The intensity, frequency, and form in which power manifests vary. Outcomes are innovative, creative, and probabilistic.

Power as a natural potential of development is neither intrinsically good nor evil. However, the form in which power manifests can be labeled constructive or destructive according to various value systems. Likewise, the repatterning can be labeled beneficial or detrimental. This theory does not value the various forms. It recognizes differences.

The literature traced the development of the ideas of power and human field motion and drew from pertinent sources to build the conception of the variables as utilized in this research. The themes of change and causality permeated the power literature. This work connected with the literature in relation to change; it departed in relation to causality. Instead, the principle of helicy postulates that change is probabilistic, innovative, and creative.[38] Acausality allows for the idea of knowing participation. The literature offered limited support for a noncausal conceptualization of power.[27, 32, 33] Further support for an acausal power theory was found in the literature on freedom, will, intentionality, and the concept of participation in quantum physics.[2, 3, 7, 8, 10–12, 14, 18, 20, 24, 25, 29, 35, 37, 41, 42, 43] The interpretation of this power theory with the literature follows:

Knowing participation is the central axiom in this theory. Power requires feeling free to act intentionally. Intentionality and will allow for imaginative participation in possibilities and spark awareness of the human capacity for change; choices demonstrate intent. No matter how limited choices may be, by means of choices humans participate in actualizing some developmental potentials rather than others. As humans are aware, they are aware that their choices make a difference in their participation in life experiences. Awareness plays a role in making choices by focusing attention on perceptions and by reflecting the flow of the organism. The spontaneous, free flow of activity and creative endeavor interplay in the human–environment interaction; this describes involvement in creating changes.

Power is the capacity to participate knowingly in change. Knowing participation is being aware of what one is choosing to do, feeling free to do it, and doing it intentionally. Awareness and freedom to act intentionally guide participation in choices and involvement in creating changes. The interrelation of the concepts of awareness, choices, freedom to act intentionally, and involvement in creating changes constitutes the theory of power whereby humans participate in innovative repatterning of the human and environmental fields. The web of relationships among the concepts arises from their synergistic relationship to the whole.

Building on Ference's development of the human field motion concept, the literature on transcendent or peak experiences and the concept of flow was explored, since HFM is postulated as an experience that transcends time and space as well as movement and stillness. Human field motion is an indicator of the continuously moving position and flow of the human field pattern. Perhaps the flow of HFM is one trigger that facilitates humans' becoming actually what they are potentially by participating knowingly in actualizing some developmental potentials rather than others. The flow of HFM is an experience of position that may facilitate power and, thus, repatterning of the human and environmental fields. The variables of HFM and power were the indicators of human change used to operationalize the principle of helicy.

METHOD

The methodological focus was of major importance in testing this theory.

The Power-as-Knowing-Participation-in-Change Test (PKPCT)

Initially, two judges' studies were conducted. Judges were selected from the nursing faculty of New York University and were considered knowledgeable in the Rogerian framework. A different form was developed for each study; each form consisted of three parts. As a result of ratings by the nine judges, semantic differential technique was utilized to construct the pilot power measure comprised of 4 concepts, 3 contexts, and 24 scales. The concepts were different field behaviors that characterized power. The contexts represented the human and environmental fields. The scales were bipolar adjective descriptors that further specified the field behaviors that characterized power. The scales included nine reference scales[17, 34] that previously had loaded, three per factor, on the factors of Evaluation (E), Potency (P), and Activity (A). A different scale selected from the pool of 24 scales appeared twice on the list of scales for each of the 12 concept–context combinations. These scales constituted retest reliability items.

Pilot Study

Usable data from a national sample of men and women ($N = 267$; response rate $= 53$ percent) representing various ages, marital, educational, and occupational backgrounds were collected. Subjects solicited from national conferences, meetings, workshops, student and colleague groups were given or mailed a packet of materials that included a cover letter, consent form, Background Information Form, Human Field Motion Test, and PKPCT.

In the pilot study for this investigation ($N = 266$), the human field motion concepts of "my motor is running" (MR) and "my field expansion"(FE) were initially factor analyzed together and loaded on different factors. This provided evidence of construct validity by supporting the theoretical position that MR and FE are two different HFM concepts. Next, MR and FE were factored separately, and the factor scores provided the basis for a new scoring method. Varimax rotation of principal factors was utilized in both instances. As a result of the pilot work, MR and FE constituted different variables in the set of HFM measures in the final study.

When the responses for each subject were strung out in a single matrix and factor analyzed utilizing principal factors with varimax rotation, three factors with eigenvalues greater than 1.0 emerged.[22, 26] Lack of simple structure suggested that, while the factors were statistically orthogonal, they described several related aspects of one constuct rather than comprising relatively distinct dimensions of power.

The reference scales did not serve as marker scales by loading on three different factors. Rather, each factor consisted of a composite of EPA scales. This phenomenon of concept–scale interaction may indicate methodological artifacts.[15] Perhaps, however, the composite clusters of EPA scales on each factor suggested the notion of different unitary, rather than particulate, dimensions of power. Could it be that the felt, cognizant activity of power, represented by the EPA scales, is empirically demonstrated by the clustering of these scales on the same factor(s)? This idea was perhaps supported by the clustering of the reference scales on a single factor when the nine reference scales were factored separately. Also, various tests for congruence indicated that power is a single dimension both in terms of contexts ("myself," "family," "occupation," which were indices of the human and environmental fields) and concepts ("awareness," "choices," "freedom to act intentionally," "involvement in creating changes"), which were field manifestations that characterize power.

Factor score means were examined in order to select those concept–context combinations that distinctly measured the most highly discriminating aspects of the underlying dimensions of power. For the revised instrument, six concept–context combinations were selected. Scales were reduced from 24 to 12; scales that loaded simultaneously on more than one factor or that did not load on any factor were eliminated.

Reliability, reported as the variances of the factor scores, ranged from 0.55 to 0.99 for the PKPCT and 0.69 to 0.81 for the HFMT. Item retest reliability ranged from 0.60 to 0.90 for the PKPCT and 0.70 to 0.82 for the HFMT. The loadings of the scales for each of the factors were the validity coefficients for measuring that factor. Validity coefficients for the PKPCT ranged from 0.51 to 0.78; the range for the HFMT was 0.42 to 0.79.

Design

This descriptive investigation utilized canonical correlation design to examine the relations between two sets of variables. The first set consisted of the human field motion measures; the second set consisted of the power measures. Canonical correlation analysis (CA) can be appropriately utilized to explore theoretical problems about content relations; it answers questions about the number and nature of mutually independent relationships between two sets of data.[6]

A volunteer national sample of adult men and women ($N = 625$) was solicited through names obtained from national association mailing lists (48 percent) or membership directories (13 percent), and groups accessible to the investigator or colleagues (38 percent). Materials were mailed to subjects, and 61 percent returned usable materials by prepaid mail. Each subject completed a consent form, the Background Information Form, the HFMT, and the PKPCT.

The sample was diverse in terms of age, sex, marital status, city size, geographical residence, education, and occupation. Fifty-five percent were women, and 45 percent were men. Ages ranged from 21 to 60, with a median age of 35. Sixty-five percent were married. The median educational level was the bachelor's degree. Fifty-one percent lived in rural communities (less than 70,000 population), and 49 percent lived in urban areas. All 50 states and Washington, D.C., were represented. Twelve occupational groups as well as a miscellaneous occupational category were included; the professions were overrepresented, and skilled and unskilled occupations were underrepresented.

RESULTS

Human Field Motion

The theoretical position that MR and FE are two different HFM concepts was again supported when the scales were initially factor analyzed together and loaded on different factors. Subsequently, MR and FE were factor analyzed as separate constructs.

The evidence for determining the number of HFM factors was not clearly demonstrated. Consequently, considering that the second factors on MR and FE had eigenvalues exceeding 1.0, and that interpretation supported the use of two factors, it was decided to proceed with two factors for each of the HFM concepts. However, the scree-test did not provide clear-cut support for selecting two factors.[19] Also, only two scales, rather than the desirable minimum of three, loaded on the second factor for both MR and FE.[19, 40] Consequently, the second factors for both MR and FE were weak.

For both MR and FE the first factor was a dynamism factor, which combines potency and activity scales, and the second factor was an evaluation factor.[34] The MR factors were named dynamic rhythmicity (DR) and imaginative vision (IV). The FE factors were named dynamic expansion (DE) and flow experience (FX). Reliability, reported as the variances of the factor scores, ranged from 0.43 to 0.87. Item retest reliability was 0.73 (FE) and 0.82 (MR). Validity coefficients, as measured by the factor loadings, ranged from 0.42 to 0.77.

Power

When data were strung out in a single matrix, one factor with an eigenvalue greater than 1.0 emerged.[22, 26] Next, the data were analyzed by subsets. The first subset was utilized for hypothesis testing. The four *concepts* along with the associated *contexts* that had demonstrated in the pilot study greater ability to measure discriminating aspects of the concepts were factor analyzed. Forty-three percent of the variance was accounted for by the only viable factor that emerged when data were strung out in a single matrix. Varimax rotation revealed that all scales loaded on this factor (0.56–0.70) named unitary power (UP). Unitary power has a valuable, intentional, important, pleasant, and orderly quality; the strength is profound, informed, assertive, expanding and is accompanied by activity that is leading, free, and seeking. Reliabilities, variances of the factor scores, for the four concept–contexts measuring power ranged from 0.63–0.99. Validity coefficients, factor loadings, ranged from 0.56–0.70.

The second subset of data was analyzed to test for further validation of congruence of the human and environmental fields. Similarity of factor structures and congruence coefficients (0.99) indicated that power, as measured by the concept of "involvement in creating changes," generalized across the contexts of "myself," "family," and "occupation." In other words, subjects did not respond in a substantially different manner when the concept was considered in relation to indicators of human and environmental fields. In the pilot and final studies, power generalized across contexts. A beginning verification of the Rogerian principle that the human and environmental fields are integral with each other was empirically demonstrated.

Treatment of the Data

Factor scores were computed for the human field motion and power variables. The HFM set consisted of DR, IV, DE, and FX. The power set consisted of "awareness in relation to occupation" (AO), "choices in relation to myself" (CS), "freedom to act intentionally in relations with family" (FF), and "involvement in creating changes in relations with family" (IF). Although only one power factor (UP) emerged, there was considerable variation among the means of the four dimensions ($\bar{x}$ = AO 0.22, CS 0.06, FF −0.03, IF −0.25) of UP. The salience of the concepts differed. Hence, factor scores for each concept represented a separate variable.

The hypothesis that there was at least one significant relationship between the set of human field motion scores and the set of concepts–contexts–scales measuring power was supported. There were two statistically significant canonical correlations of 0.61 and 0.16; the sum of the squared correlations accounted for 40 percent of shared variance.

Although the matrix of weights was used in computing the canonical correlation, the content of the variables was interpreted by means of the structure coefficients.[21] Structure coefficients are correlations of the original variables with the canonical variate.[4, 6, 21] Two of the four HFM variables contributed meaningfully to the first canonical variate (0.88, 0.93); all of the power measures contributed meaningfully (0.56, 0.70, 0.88, 0.89).

Since IV and FX, the second MR and FE factors, did not contribute substantially to the first variate (0.05, 0.34), this experiential imaginative flow was not related to the first power variate. IV and FX did load highly on the second HFM canonical variate (0.65, 0.85); yet, again, they were largely unrelated to power (R_c = 0.16), which had low loadings on the second variate. As had been theoretically described, perhaps the imaginative flow of IV and FX captures the passive receptivity dimension of HFM that is complementary to the active assertion dimension of rhythmic expansion.

Similarly to the power factor structure, the structure coefficients in the canonical analysis suggested that power was a synergistic composite of different unitary, rather than particulate, dimensions of power. Since the second canonical correlation was too low to be of substantive importance, it was neither named nor further interpreted.

Both the redundancy index and the sum of squared canonical correlations have been proposed as means of interpreting the strength of the relationship in CA.[4, 13, 16, 21, 28, 30, 31] In this study, the redundancy index for the power measures (0.37) and the redundancy index for the HFM measures (0.32) were similar to the sum of the squared canonical correlations (0.40).

Ancillary Analysis

One way analyses of variance revealed no statistically significant differences related to sex or education for the four HFM variables and the four power variables. In relation to age, analyses of variance revealed statistically significant relationships with FX, CS, FF, and IF. However, none of the correlations were ≥ 0.20. Analyses of variance revealed statistically significant relationships between occupation and FX, AO, FF, IF. Correlations ≥ 0.20 were present for AO ($r = 0.20$), FF ($r = 0.22$), and IF ($r - 0.22$).

Little is known regarding variables related to the nursing science variables of HFM and power. Therefore, items eliciting descriptive patterns were constructed and included in the Background Information Form. For the HFM variables, feeling a sense of oneness with nature was related to IV ($r - 0.15$); engagement in self-development activities was related to FX ($r = 0.15$); self-confidence was related to DR ($r = 0.21$) and DE ($r = 0.23$). For the power variables, CS was related to self-development ($r = 0.19$), hopefulness ($r = 0.15$), and self-confidence ($r = 0.28$). Self-confidence was also related to AO ($r = 0.21$) and FF ($r = 0.16$). Additional relationships were discovered among the matrix of descriptive pattern variables. However, all correlations in the descriptive pattern analysis were low.

DISCUSSION AND RECOMMENDATIONS

Power, a continuous theme in the flow of life experiences, was investigated to enhance understanding of unitary human beings, the phenomenon of concern to the discipline of nursing. Support of the hypothesis suggested that as HFM, an index of unitary human development, proceeds, so does the capacity to participate knowingly. Higher-frequency power was related to the human field whose development appeared to have evolved further in the direction of accelerated HFM. Perhaps to change is to be in motion and have power. The rhythmic spontaneity of HFM contrasts with, but is complementary to, the deliberate knowing participation of power. Ference[9] indicated that HFM may be similar to flow experience, peak experience, and timeless experience and noted that her findings suggested a four-dimensional space–time quality of HFM. In this study, the structure coefficients of IV and FX on the second HFM canonical variate would seem to support the view that the flow of HFM is an experience that transcends space and time as well as movement and stillness.

Maslow[23] noted that peak experiences suggested a paradox in that rational, logical aspects coexisted with the symbolic, metaphorical, and unexplainable qualities of the experience. Similarly, HFM suggests a paradox. The first factors described MR and FE as clear, wakeful, bright, and active, in contrast with the imaginative, visionary, boundaryless qualities of the second factors. The high structure coefficients of the second HFM factors on the second canonical variate also indicated measurement of different manifestations of MR and FE. In future studies the addition of evaluation scales might increase the reliability of the second

MR and FE factors and allow for more adequate measurement of the four-dimensional space–time quality of HFM.

While one viable factor emerged from the power data, factor score means demonstrated that the operationalized salience of each power concept was different. Perhaps "involvement in creating changes" requires the feeling of "freedom to act intentionally," which in turn may be related to the kind of "choices" one makes. It would seem that the relationships are consistent even when "awareness" is present. The explanation for the clustering of EPA scales on one factor is unclear. The loading of all the scales on one factor was theoretically consistent. However, homogeneous concept selection provides an alternate methodological explanation.[15] Perhaps measurement of the power concepts by a different methodological approach, such as multidimensional scaling or the Likert scaling technique, might define more precisely the nature of the differences among the power concepts.

Findings from the ancillary analyses suggest possible tendencies rather than precise measurements. A majority (69 percent) considered what happened in their lives to be primarily related to a mutual interaction of themselves and their environment rather than "forces" inside (25 percent) or outside (6 percent) their "control." Likewise, did subjects perceive themselves as unitary rather than dichotomous when 60 percent reported that they were equally intuitive and rational rather than one (20 percent) or the other (20 percent)? Perhaps the relationship of IV and FX to having experienced a sense of oneness with nature provides some clues for further understanding the nature of these second factors of MR and FE. Also, the matrix of relationships among subjects' descriptive patterns suggested pattern changes that may generate ideas for further research. Is the meditation–less sleep relationship indicative of a high-frequency pattern characterizing evolutionary emergence? Does the relationship of having had peak experiences and a sense of timelessness to having also experienced a sense of oneness with nature provide further evidence of the nature and direction of unitary human development?

Few statistically significant differences among relevant demographic variables and HFM or power were discovered. Most importantly, the findings verified the theoretical perspectives that age and sex are not meaningful predictors of HFM and power. In future studies, the issue of chronological age needs to be examined more critically.

The ubiquity of power emphasizes the importance of a nursing theory that enhances the understanding of unitary human beings in continuous mutual process with the environment. In light of implications for education, practice, and research, specific recommendations for further research are offered:

1. Replicate this study with careful attention to selecting a sample that is representative of the diversity of American society. The relationships of age, sex, education, and occupation to power need to be examined more critically. Controlling for length of service, a comparison of achievement and scope of responsibility within and among occupations could also be investigated. Breakdown of equal-sized groups by age, sex, education, and oc-

cupation might identify clustering of high frequency power in particular groups. Subsequently, known-groups technique could be used for construct validation of the power instrument. The methodology could be strengthened by: (a) increasing the response rate; (b) collecting the data in a standardized manner; (c) improving the measurement of human field motion and power

2. Knowledgeable, meaningful participation in the repatterning process has implications for the nursing profession and clinical practice. Translation of the theory to a model that can be tested in education and practice is a future step. The relationship of the registered professional nurse's power pattern and whether or not this facilitates further development of power in clients could be explored. The PKPCT can also be utilized as an assessment and teaching device with clients to enhance understanding of their continuous, mutual process with the environment

3. The theory described the phenomenon of power as the capacity to participate knowingly in change and indicated that the way one knowingly participates can manifest in a diversity of forms. This study focused on the phenomenon of power. Research investigating particular power *forms* that characterize how one knowingly participates is needed

4. This study was limited to the investigation of power as a human field manifestation perceived in relation to the human and environmental fields. It is suggested that power be examined from the perspective of the environmental field or the two fields in interaction. Formal testing of hypotheses derived from the principle of integrality is required to further support the proposition that, while the two fields are by definition different, they are integral with one another

5. Integration of the helicy studies,[1, 5, 36] accompanied by a review of the change literature to delineate similarities and differences with helicy, might result in theoretically based testable theorems that could account for additional variance of power

6. Further theoretically based methodological development of the HFMT and PKPCT is indicated. Specific recommendations were previously presented

7. Investigation of the relationship of hope, confidence, and self-development to power is suggested. Also, predictors of power from other frameworks, if reconceptualized within a new world view, might prove fruitful in relation to power as described in this research

8. The relationship of indicators of rhythmicity, such as meditation, flow experiences, timelessness, a sense of oneness with the universe, and joy, to human field motion could be explored

The unitary human being is the central focus of the discipline of nursing. This study, through the development and testing of a new power theory, provided a beginning search for answers to Rogers' question concerning the capacity of human beings to repattern the human and environmental fields.[38]

REFERENCES

1. Barrett EAM: An Empirical Investigation of Martha E. Rogers' Principle of Helicy: The Relationship of Human Field Motion and Power, doctoral dissertation. New York University, 1983 (University Microfilms Publication No: 84-06, 278)
2. Bugental JFT: The Search for Authenticity. New York, Holt, Rinehart & Winston, 1965
3. Capra F: The Tao of Physics. Berkeley, Shambhala, 1975
4. Cooley WW, Lohnes PR: Multivariate Data Analysis. New York, Wiley, 1971
5. Cowling WR III: The Relationship of Mystical Experience, Differentiation, and Creativity in College Students: An Empirical Investigation of the Principle of Helicy in Rogers' Science of Unitary Human Beings, doctoral dissertation. New York University, 1983 (University Microfilms Publication No:84-06, 283)
6. Darlington R, Weinberg S, Walberg H: In Amick D, Walberg H (eds): Introductory Multivariate Analysis. Berkeley, McCutcheon Publishing, 1975
7. Dubos R: A God Within. New York, Scribner's, 1972
8. Dubos R: Interview: Rene Dubos. Omni 2 (3):87–88; 126; 128, 1979
9. Ference HM: The Relationship of Time Experience, Creativity Traits, Differentiation, and Human Field Motion: An Empirical Investigation of Rogers' Correlates of Synergistic Human Development, doctoral dissertation. New York University, 1979 (University Microfilms Publication No:80-10, 281)
10. Ferguson M: The Aquarian Conspiracy. Los Angeles, Tarcher, 1980
11. Ford DH, Urban HB: Systems of Psychotherapy. New York, Wiley, 1963
12. Frankl VE: The Will to Meaning. New York, New American Library, 1969
13. Gleason TC: On redundancy in canonical analysis. Psychol Bull 83:1004–1006, 1976
14. Guardini R: Power and Responsibility. Chicago, Regnery, 1961
15. Heise DR: Some methodological issues in semantic differential research. Psychol Bull 72:406–422, 1969
16. Holland TR, Levi M, Watson, CG: Canonical correlation in the analysis of a contingency table. Psychol Bull 87:334–336, 1980
17. Jakobovits LA: Comparative psycholinguistics in the study of cultures. Int J Psychol 1:15–37, 1966
18. James W: The Principles of Psychology, Vol 2. New York, Dover, 1950 (Originally published 1890)
19. Kim J, Mueller CW: Factor analysis: Statistical methods and practical issues. In Sullivan JL (ed): Series: Quantitative Applications in the Social Sciences, Series No. 07–014. Beverly Hills, Sage 1978
20. Knight RP: Determinism, "freedom," and psychotherapy. Psychiatry 9:251–262, 1946
21. Levine MS: Canonical Analysis and Factor Comparison. Beverly Hills, Sage, 1977
22. Maguire TO: Semantic differential methodology for the structuring of attitudes. Am Ed Res J 10:295–306, 1973
23. Maslow AH: Comments on Dr. Frankl's paper. J Humanistic Psych 6:107–112, 1966
24. May R: Love and Will. New York, Dell, 1969
25. May R: Power and Innocence. New York, Dell, 1972
26. Mayerberg CK, Bean AG: Two types of factors in the analysis of semantic differential attitude data. Applied Psychological Measurement 2:469–480, 1978
27. McClusky JE: Power without control: Exemplary power. Paper presented at the annual meeting of the American Political Science Association, St. Louis, September 1975

28. Miller JK: The Development and Application of Bi-Multivariate Correlation: A Measure of Statistical Association Between Multivariate Measurement Sets, doctoral dissertation. State University of New York at Buffalo, 1969
29. Muller HJ: Freedom as the ability to choose and carry out purposes. In Freedom: Its History, Nature and Varieties. London, Macmillan, 1970
30. Nicewander WA, Wood DA: Comments on "A general canonical correlation index." Psychol Bull 81:92–94, 1974
31. Nie NH, Hull CH, Jenkins JG, Steinbrenner J, Bent DH: SPSS: Statistical Package for the Social Sciences, 2nd ed. New York, McGraw-Hill, 1975
32. Nietzsche F: The Will to Power. Kaufmann E ed and trans, & Hollingdale RJ, trans. New York, Random House, 1969 (Original notes 1883–1888)
33. Olsen ME: Power as a social process. In Olsen ME (ed): Power in Societies. New York, Macmillan, 1970
34. Osgood CE, Suci CJ, Tannenbaum PH: The Measurement of Meaning. Chicago, University of Illinois Press, 1957
35. Parsons HL: A definition of freedom. Main Currents Mod Thought 10:57–60, 1954
36. Raile MM: The Relationships of Creativity, Actualization, and Empathy in Unitary Human Development: A Descriptive Study of M. Rogers' Principle of Helicy, doctoral dissertation. New York University, 1983 (University Microfilms Publication No: 83-13, 874)
37. Rogers C: Carl Rogers on Personal Power. New York, Delacorte Press, 1977
38. Rogers ME: An Introduction to the Theoretical Basis of Nursing. Philadelphia, FA Davis, 1970
39. Rogers ME: Nursing science: A science of unitary man, terminology, New York University Division of Nursing, April 1, 1981 (unpublished)
40. Thurstone LL: Multiple-Factor Analysis. Chicago, University of Chicago Press, 1947
41. Wheeler JA Thorne KS, Misner C: Gravitation. San Francisco, W.A. Freeman, 1973
42. Wheelis A: How People Change. New York, Harper Colophon Books, 1975
43. Zukav G: The Dancing Wu-Li Masters. New York, Morrow, 1979

Critique of Barrett's Study

Joyce J. Fitzpatrick

Barrett concerned her research with the principle of helicy through a study of the relationship between human field motion and power. She further delineated the power concept into four components and discussed these in relation to Rogers' conceptualization. An additional concern of this investigator was the development of an instrument to measure power and evaluation of the validity and reliability of this measurement.

Barrett's research was clearly based on the work of Ference. This study, in addition, provided a good illustration of extension of previous research. Barrett devised a new scoring method for the Human Field Motion Test. This should be further assessed in relation to the previous scoring method. Such continued refinement of instruments will assist in clarification of the components of major interest in expanding the knowledge base related to Rogers.

As noted by Barrett, the previous literature included limited support for a noncausal conceptualization of power. Barrett has contributed in the extension of the knowledge base and in the conceptualization of power as the capacity to participate knowingly in change.

Barrett did include some sweeping generalizations in her descriptions that were not warranted, both in relation to the conceptualization leading to this study and the interpretation of results. As theoretical links are more tightly developed, such will be omitted necessarily. This will add strength to the research.

In summary, Barrett has creatively approached development of Rogers' conceptualization in relation to the concept of power, a new approach, and extended the study of human field motion. A strong base was provided for extending this research.

Response

Elizabeth Ann Manhart Barrett

Helicy concerns the nature and direction of change. In this theoretical and methodological study, the human field motion and power variables were the indicators of human change used to operationalize the principle of helicy. The theory explicated the relationship of measures indicative of the direction of change (human field motion variables) and measures indicative of the nature of change (power variables). It is suggested that serious readers refer to the original work to more adequately critique the theoretical linkages, the empirical testing, and the interpretation of findings (*An Empirical Investigation of Martha E. Rogers' Principle of Helicy: The Relationship of Human Field Motion and Power*. University Microfilms No: 84–06278).

Fitzpatrick makes a crucial point: The research will be strengthened as the conceptual links become more fully delineated and as findings accumulate. This is perhaps the most difficult and most important challenge in initial stages of research. This study was a beginning attempt to conceptualize and measure power from a Rogerian view. In addition, building on Ference's research, the human field motion concept was further delineated. As Fitzpatrick noted, future researchers are invited to assess the new scoring in relation to Ference's scoring method for the Human Field Motion Test. Additionally, many exciting possibilities for derivation of testable theorems concerning human field motion and power have potential for expanding the knowledge base of human development in the Science of Unitary Human Beings.

Critique of Barrett's Study

Helen M. Ference

Barrett's study of 1983 is a landmark study in the Science of Unitary Human Beings. The beginning thoughts and theoretical derivations of this work actually began in the late seventies, when there was an explosion of terminology development in Rogers' framework. These study findings support the principle of helicy. Specifically, there is a relationship between human field motion and power. As the human energy field evolves in the direction of increased frequency and more differentiation of pattern and organization, man's ability to participate knowingly also increases. The power tool developed through this research measures the knowing participation of change of the human energy field.

Prior to this study, the only tool (instrument) developed to measure four-dimensional man was Ference's Human Field Motion Test. Barrett developed the Power-as-Knowing-Participation-in-Change Test (PKPCT) as a measure of the connotative meaning of feelings, in this case, the "freedom-to-act-intentionally" feeling. Barrett discusses the construct of power as a natural potential in all human beings. Future researchers and writers should be cautious not to assign a positive or negative value to this power, especially during the early stages of research. The verification of Rogers' principles of resonancy and helicy, by the positive relationship between motion and power, marks a promising future for ongoing tool development and refinement of theories in the Science of Unitary Human Beings.

Barrett's use of factor analysis techniques to explain meaningful relationships among the power and motion variable sets is exceptional. The use of canonical correlation as an exploration technique is well suited for investigating within this framework. This technique utilizes the process of synthesis to identify significant multidimensions for the yet unnamed constructs. It becomes imperative, as findings unfold in this new science, that we adhere to the terminology of previous researchers until we can logically or empirically provide new terms or redefinitions. Barrett offers new terms, such as "dynamic rhythmicity" and "imaginative vision," to the newly found factors of human field motion. She then correlates these new variables with those explaining the power construct. Her description of this process, while highly technical, is essential to comprehending the nature of change as theoretically presented.

A most interesting, secondary finding is noteworthy. Barrett originally set up the scales of the power tool to be rated against concepts in the three different contexts of (1) myself, (2) the family, and (3) the occupation. She finds no difference in the ratings across these three contexts in her study population. Of course, this finding supports the principle of complementarity, that the human and environmental energy fields are in continuous mutual process. However, could we speculate that there might be differences across these contextual frameworks—for persons described as having multiple personalities, for example? Perhaps an investigation of this special subpopulation, using the original power tool, would lead to an understanding of multiple manifestations and the meaning of the human energy field.

Another interesting finding reported by Barrett is that chronological age is not a predictor of human field motion or power. This finding suggests that the human energy field may be more or less evolved in space–time, unrelated to linear time. Future researchers, however, should be cautious about the chronological age selections for study subjects, since the tools measuring power and motion have the three-dimensional handicap of showing scale-checking differences over the chronological age of 60.

In summary, Barrett has conducted one of the largest known studies ($N = 625$) in the Science of Unitary Human Beings. Although she used a volunteer sample, it was diverse. It seems unlikely that a random sample would respond much differently. However, if this study is replicated (as Barrett requests), a national, random sample is preferred. Barrett has made an important contribution to our understanding of the nature of change in unitary man. Once we begin to operationalize the meaning of the factors described, our nursing practice may vary. For example, is the "experiential, imaginative flow" (that does not correlate with power) an attribute that is necessary for maintaining the human field pattern and organization at a lesser frequency? Might we find a correlation between "experiential, imaginative flow" and power (or a lack of "experiential, imaginative flow") in subpopulations experiencing energy field transitions, such as dying, battering, or loss of function? This study opens the door for many new areas for investigation within this science. Barrett describes the construct of power for the first time in a four-dimensional perspective and provides a beginning tool for future investigation.

Response
Elizabeth Ann Manhart Barrett

Second only to Rogers, Ference's work formed the basis for this beginning research. In addition to the evolution of thought that flowed from Ference's theoretical formulations, the demonstration of the usefulness of semantic differential technique in concretizing the abstract notions of the Rogerian conceptual system and canonical correlation analysis as an exploratory technique that provides information concerning many-to-many patterns of association are pragmatic examples.

Ference's critique suggests a beginning dialogue that may guide future investigations and perhaps foster translation of the theory to a model that can be tested in education and clinical practice. While speculative, as Ference noted, such discussion may prove useful in stimulating development of necessary conceptual linkages, theory derivation, and hypothesis generation. Specifically, Ference offers a fresh view of the findings regarding the second factors of human field motion and suggests that operationalizing the meaning of the factors may have implications for nursing practice. Ference ponders the idea that experiential, imaginative flow may be "an attribute that is necessary for maintaining the human field pattern at a lesser frequency." Or might experiential, imaginative flow characterize a higher frequency human field pattern as manifest by experiences that seem timeless, motionless? Would a subpopulation experiencing burnout manifest lower frequency experiential imaginative flow, dynamic rhythmicity, and power?

Ference cautions future researchers and writers not to assign a positive or negative value to the power phenomenon. This will be especially crucial in delineation of the *forms* in which power manifests, as well as the conceptualization of power in relation to the mutual process of the human and environmental fields.

Afterword

Violet M. Malinski

This book was designed to stimulate a collegial exchange of ideas. Researchers exploring the Science of Unitary Human Beings share common problems and can benefit from others' experiences. Of the eight studies presented, two produced tools developed within this conceptual system, a valuable resource for future investigators. Ference developed and tested the Human Field Motion Test, later used by Gueldner and refined by Barrett, who also developed and tested a set of scales to assess Power-as-Knowing-Participation-in-Change. Multiple explorations of such variables as time experience, creativity, differentiation, lightwaves, and human field motion contribute to the growth of a body of information that can serve as a springboard for future work.

Moving away from the linear, sequential perspective of traditional science with its focus on causality, we find ourselves dealing with variables that are integral to an underlying process rather than discrete, isolated events. The relationships between observer and observed and between aspects of a process that become manifest and those that are "hidden" are crucial to any investigation. Taking an example from quantum mechanics (the world of fundamental particles), there are conjugate variables, integral pairs (e.g., momentum and position of a particle) whose shared symmetry describes a process that cannot be explained except by their interaction.[8] Thus a number of studies presented used correlational designs with independent and dependent variables designed not to imply a causal relationship but, as Cowling expressed it, to describe patterned mutual change.

The unitary human being's direct experiencing of the mutual process of field interaction is a unifying theme across the studies presented. Reeder suggests the phenomenological philosophy of science as an alternative to the logical-empiricist approach of deducing hypotheses, checking the system for internal consistency, and looking for correspondence to the external world.[7] The phenomenological approach would assist with research into the integral interaction between the knower and the known in which, for example, one would examine ''colors as imagined'' rather than color preference as the variable under consideration.[7] In this way the human and environmental field interaction can be studied as the unitary process it is, permitting testing of this conceptual system through examination of relationships among phenomena that evolve from the interaction (mutual patterned change). Reeder sees phenomenology as a step toward developing ''wave seeing'' rather than ''particle seeing,'' thus helping us develop the ''pattern seeing of wave phenomena'' so important to research within Rogers' system.[7]

Newman also identified a methodology of pattern as appropriate to the development of nursing knowledge in general.[4] She highlighted the contradiction between traditional research methodology grounded in the scientific method, which is context-stripping, and the focus of nursing inquiry, human experience, which is context-dependent. In calling for alternative methodologies, both qualitative and quantitative, she joins a growing number of nurses.[1-3, 5, 6, 9-11]

One of the difficulties in developing this pattern is seeing that we are dealing with interconnections that do not manifest themselves in ways accessible to the senses, as with traditional forms of data. Grasping the patterning of the whole implicitly, as a single wave (see Chapter 2) often seems to require a leap of faith. Again, borrowing an example from quantum mechanics, fundamental particles are indistinguishable; only when they leave a record on a physicist's measuring apparatus can he or she observe them.[8] Human perception of this record from the subatomic world takes place in the realm of classical physics (see discussion in Chapter 3). Still, the physicist cannot claim to have seen a particle; what is left is an approximation, a rough measure of a quantum event. Even with further tool development and refinement in this conceptual system, researchers have, at best, only rough measures at their disposal.

Interest in Rogers' Science of Unitary Human Beings is growing, and this interest is not limited to any one school or region of the country. In 1981, for example, a symposium on research related to the system was presented as part of the conference held by the American Nurses' Association Council of Nurse Researchers. The speakers were doctoral candidates at Wayne State University in Detroit, Michigan. At the First National Rogerian Conference sponsored by the Division of Nursing at New York University in 1983, participants came from across this country and Canada. Rogers receives letters and requests for information from the international community, as well. The contributors to this book hope that by sharing information with colleagues we can facilitate efforts at networking.

REFERENCES

1. Aamodt A: Examining ethnography for nurse researchers. West J Nurs Res 4:209–221, 1982
2. Gulino CK: Entering the mysterious dimension of the other: An existentialist approach to nursing care. Nurs Outlook 30: 352–357, 1982

3. Munhall PL: Nursing philosophy and nursing research: In apposition or opposition? Nurs Res 3:176–177, 181, 1982
4. Newman MA: Editorial. Adv in Nurs Sci 2:x–xi, 1983
5. Oiler C: The phenomenological approach in nursing research. Nurs Res 31:178–181, 1982
6. Omery A: Phenomenology: A method for nursing research. Adv in Nurs Sci 5:49–63, 1983
7. Reeder F: Philosophical issues in the Rogerian science of unitary human beings. Adv in Nurs Sci 6:14–23, 1984
8. Rohrlich F: Facing quantum mechanical reality. Science 221:1251–1255, 23 September 1983
9. Swanson JM, Chenitz WC: Why qualitative research in nursing? Nurs Outlook 30:241–245, 1982
10. Tinkle MB, Beaton JL: Toward a new view of science: Implications for nursing research. Adv in Nurs Sci 5:27–36, January, 1983
11. Wilson LM, Fitzpatrick JJ: Dialectic thinking as a means of understanding systems-in-development: Relevance to Rogers' principles. Adv in Nurs Sci 6:24–41, 1984

Selected Definitions

The following terms have been defined by Rogers or by those working within the system. For words that do not have specific definitions within the Science of Unitary Human Beings, the reader is referred to the general language definition as found in a dictionary.

Art.* The imaginative and creative use of knowledge.

Change. The process of becoming more differentiated and diverse in patterning.

Conceptual System.* An abstraction. A representation of the universe or some portion thereof.

Energy Field.* The fundamental unit of the living and the nonliving. "Field" is a unifying concept. "Energy" signifies the dynamic nature of the field. Energy fields are infinite.

Environment (Environmental Field).* An irreducible, four-dimensional energy field identified by patterning and integral with the human field.

Four-Dimensional. Reality perceived as a synthesis of nonlinear coordinates from which innovative change continuously and evolutionarily emerges (Rogers, 1978). A nonlinear domain without spatial or temporal attributes (Rogers, 1982)

---

*Taken from Rogers ME: *Nursing science: A science of unitary human beings, glosssary*. Unpublished paper, New York University, 1982.

Human Field Motion. The experience of the continuous moving flow of human field patterning as measured by Ference's (1979) Human Field Motion Test. This experience is measured by bipolar adjective scales that rate the meaning of "my motor is running" and "my field expansion."

Learned Profession.* A science and an art.

Negentropy.* Increasing heterogeneity, differentiation, diversity, complexity of patterning.

Nursing. A learned profession (see definition of "learned profession"). The science, the organized body of abstract knowledge which serves as the theoretical basis for the profession, focuses on unitary human beings integral with the environment and is unique to nursing. The art involves the creative use of this knowledge to serve humanity.

Patterning.* The distinguishing characteristic of an energy field perceived as a single wave.

Power.* The capacity to participate knowingly in the process of change. Power is measured by the Power-as-Knowing-Participation-in-Change Test, in which the semantic differential technique is used to rate "awareness," "choices," "freedom to act intentionally," and "involvement in creating changes" in relation to self, family, and occupation (Barrett, 1983).

Principles of Homeodynamics. Developed from the conceptual system of the Science of Unitary Human Beings. Together they describe the nature and direction of change manifested by unitary human beings in mutual process with the environment. These principles are:

> **Principle of Resonancy.** The continuous change from lower to higher frequency wave patterns in human and environmental fields.

> **Principle of Helicy.** The continuous, innovative, probabilistic increasing diversity of human and environmental field patterns characterized by non-repeating rhythmicities.

> **Principle of Integrality.** The continuous mutual human field and environmental field process.

Science.* An organized body of abstract knowledge arrived at by scientific research and logical analysis.

Unitary Human Being (Human Field).* An irreducible, four-dimensional energy field identified by patterning and manifesting characteristics that are specific to the whole and cannot be predicted from knowledge of the parts.

Wave. An oscillating manifestation of the human energy field, proposed to be an index of unitary human beings (Ference, 1979).

Index

Italicized page numbers refer to figures. Italic *n* after page numbers refers to footnotes.